Chinese Medication

Unlock the Power of Chinese Herbs

(Essential Guide to Nutritional Remedies to Restore Wellness of the Body System)

Robert Hansen

Published By **Bella Frost**

Robert Hansen

Chinese Medication: Unlock the Power of Chinese Herbs (Essential Guide to Nutritional Remedies to Restore Wellness of the Body System)

ISBN 978-1-9994868-2-2

Legal & Disclaimer

Table Of Contents

Chapter 1: Basic and Fundamental Chemistry

What exactly is the human body? The human body is comprised of around 37 trillion cells and more than 100 trillion of bacteria! From to the highest point of our heads all the way to the soles of our feet, there are nothing more than chemical reactions happening. The human body is composed from 50 to 75 of water. A majority of the water that is in our bodies is found inside the cells of our bodies. Knowing this is essential for all human beings. Each organ of our body is nothing more than a group of cells serving an exact function and come together like a huge puzzle. If you're looking at your heart or hair, the liver or prostate, they're all one of the cells. Nature isn't random and everything happens using God-given intelligence human beings will never be able to fully grasp. Like every other living thing living on earth cells consume energy to fuel their bodies and expels garbage. The waste is the result from a chemical reaction for instance (industrial waste or biological waste, as well as pollution from the atmosphere). It is why people consume food and have to provide trillions and trillions of cells starting from the moment they're born until the day they die. The primary reason why illness is evident is due to the body's inability to clean rid of the cell and bodily wastes. It is a literal breakdown into dis (meaning absence of) and ease (meaning physical comfort and a relaxed state in your body). The term "disease" refers to something that is physical and not circulating within the body. The answer is obvious to the question of what this physical thing is: waste! In the average, from mouth to anus is about 30 feet. This is how much food needs to travel within the body before it is and digested. It takes between 6 and 8 hours to get into the small intestines by itself. In order to fully digest food, the time can take between 12 and 16 hours. One of the problems with Americans is their consistency and excessive consumption of their food. If you are eating 3 meals daily and two meals for the next 60 years think about how much trash is accumulating and stored within the body. It's a simple math, lets say that it takes you 12 hours to take in your food completely. Then, you eat three meals per day, with not snack, which is 123=36. The human body only has 24 hours in a single day and, in the theory of things it will take minimum 1.5 days for you to be able to digest the 3 meals that you had eaten the day before and not eating food for the day. We can now see how the accumulation of waste in time takes place. If the person who was ill continued to do in the same way for more than 60 years, then disease as well as other ailments are an absolute. In the average, the human body from the mouth to the anus is joined by a 30 foot or 9 meters of tube. In comparison this is the equivalent of four

Shaquille Of Neil (7'1 feet) perched on top of each the other! It's quite a distance to journey after each dinner. This is why many people feel sluggish and fatigued after having an enormous, unhealthy dinner. Your body must do lots of work in order to deal with all that has consumed. In Physics we define Work is the term used to describe the transfer of energy that occurs whenever an object is moved across a long distance due to the external force part of it is acted upon to the direction of the first displacement. According to that definition, every time eating, we need to be aware of the amount of effort we're causing the body to do.

Minerals that make up the human body

One of my top Quotes from all time is from Linus Pauling. Who exactly is Linus Pauling you think? He was among four individuals throughout History who were awarded two Nobel Prizes for the area of Science. He claimed that "you can connect every sickness each disease, illness and health problem to a mineral deficit". The quote alone can show how crucial minerals are for the body. An examination of western medicine method is Genomics come first followed by neurotransmitters and hormones, then enzymes, and then Vitamins. It is a problem that minerals are seldom discussed. Vitamins will not work within the body if there's no any minerals in the body. This is like having a vehicle running without a source of energy to drive it. Minerals need to be present in order to allow vitamins to perform their functions. When a Vitamin performs its job is known as a co-enzyme. A vitamin is or amino acid and mineral, working in tandem to create something. There aren't any minerals which means there's none of the vitamins which work to become enzymes. The hormones and neurotransmitters produced through enzymes. Without minerals, that means there are no vitamins which convert to enzymes that make hormones as well as neurotransmitters. In addition, genes are saturated with nutrients, minerals and enzymes, from the time your birth until when you die. Minerals form the basis of all metabolic processes inside the body. This is why it's important to understand which and how many nutrients our body requires for optimal functioning and maintaining equilibrium.

We will look at the proportion between the minerals in our body and Earth's crust.

Elements Human Body Earth's Crust

Oxygen 65% 49%

Carbon 18% <1%

Hydrogen 10% <1%

Nitrogen 3% trace

Calcium 2% 3%

Iron <0.05% 5%

Aluminum <0.001% 8%

Silicon Trace 26%

Something to note in the graph above is the proportion to the human body, which comprises Oxygen, Carbon and Hydrogen. 93% which is almost all of the cells in your body. They run through carbon (which refers to sugar) as well as Oxygen. Carbon functions as a gas that your cells use and provides cells the energy they need to run. Oxygen acts as the ignition that allows the gas to be to be ignited. If you do not have sugars (fructose sugar, glucose or galactose) the cells you have will not be able to eat or function correctly. Galactose, galactose and fructose break into Carbon, which are the basis for Carbohydrates that are carbon chain substitutes. There are poly, simple complex, and simple carbohydrates. Simple carbohydrates comprise most fruits, and a few vegetables. Complex and poly are referred to as starch. Humans are primarily dependent on these components, particularly basic carbohydrate. The entire organic chemistry field is based upon the research of carbon chains and carbon. The human body is Carbon life forms. We absorb oxygen through the air. We then mix it with carbon on a cellular levels to create ATP (adenosine triphosphate) which provides the source of energy for all the cells. This article will look at several other important minerals found in our bodies and the functions they play.

Chromium- Sugar metabolism and cofactor for minerals

The tooth is a phosphate-based one and muscle development

Calcium-based dental and muscle development and cardiovascular health. Strong bones and teeth

Manganese- bone health

Zinc is a brain mineral cells and immune function

Potassium-blood pressure and oxygenated to the brain

Coppermetabolic process

Magnesiumregulates heart rate Relaxes muscles

Selenium- immune function

Chlorine- aids in digestion (hydrochloric acid)

Siliconbone and connective health of tissues

Skin, hair and nails

Na2+ is a component of muscle and nerve perform

The thyroid function of iodine.

Acid and Base (Alkaline)

The body prefers to live in a pH that is alkaline. The blood pH of human beings is alkaline in the normal region between 7.35 and 7.45. What is the significance of this take note of? Let's talk about some general understanding of chemistry. Chemically, there are chemical reactions which occur at all levels. A majority, if not all, reactions take place in a solution. In our case, it's the fluid in our bodies. In the event that an chemical reaction occurs, it is either gained or destroyed. As the water (H_2O) is the largest and most commonly used solution on the planet and within our bodies we measure the loss or gained Hydrogen (H) molecules by performing the test of pH. The test can range from zero to fourteen. Since water is the medium, it has a pH of 7. Anything less than 7 is deemed to range as being slightly acidic or acid. Anything over 7 is considered as being basic enough to solid base. Every one of our 37 trillion cells as well as 100 trillion bacteria are covered by the fluids of our bodies. They're referred to as interstitial fluids. One of the most well-known is obviously blood plasma. It is claims to be somewhat alkaline. It is also known as lymph fluid and tissue fluid. The blood is composed of proteins, water minerals, hormones, ions and a few other waste. Tissue Fluid is used to bathe the tissues, Similar to blood plasma, it does not contain proteins. Lymph is a tissue fluid that drains into the lymphatic system. In essence all chemical reaction that occurs between cells takes place within these fluids that regulate each aspect of the biological process in a human. The various reactions that take place are more likely to be favored within a solution that is slightly acidic.

Acidity and Alkalinity as well as their balance are the foundations of good the health. However, this is in accordance to the old saying: As Above, So Below. Our world is full that is dominated by feminine and masculine energy. There's a boundary between both, however we all need to be aware of the difference to find Peace that is basically the process of finding equilibrium. Acid is the masculine aspect of the chemistry. In science, an acid will give away its Hydrogen proton at will, and is described as a proton donor. Acids are corrosive, volatile and volatile. Acids are necessary, but using them excessive amounts can be very harmful. Like a child who would like to cut something up so that he can see the parts of it and attempt to grasp its structures. Like a toy, car, computer etc. The masculine energy is connected to the left part that controls the brain. The left brain performs tasks that require logic and logical thinking. As with math, science, and architecture. The right brain is feminine and is alkaline-based. The right-side of the brain is connected to artistic expression and creativity. It is associated with music, drawing the feeling of love and compassion. The term "base" in the field of science can be described as a proton acceptor. It means that it accepts proton acceptors Hydrogen that is released from Acid through the course of a chemical reaction. Our body, for example within the stomach we find hydrochloric acid, which has a pH range of

1-3, which in the scale of pH is very acidic. It's necessary for breaking down waste and bacteria that are present in our body. In contrast there is the Pancreas gland that makes up the lymphatic system, creates sodium bicarbonate within the body to neutralize the effects of acid. It ranges between 7.2 and 8.2 pH. The pH for normal skin ranges from 5.5 which makes it acidic. The body is always finding ways to achieve tranquility, equilibrium and peace. The saliva we breath as well as throughout our body has 7.1 or 7.5 pH for a healthy individual, which makes it somewhat alkaline. This means that when we place an acidic substance into our body, that isn't out of nature, there is a conflict. Chemicals are the basis of every activity in our existence. As we move into time we discover that we were mostly alkaline-based. Fruits, berries as well as some vegetables in the majority of cases until our diets changed to an ACID base. The main ingredient of the Acid basis diet are discomfort and inflammation. The presence of unnatural acids inside the body has an immediate result of the consumption of foods that are high in acidity as well as an increase in inflammation. What constitutes as an Acid creating food? Animal products of all kinds, animals by-products, the majority of grain, legumes in general, and some even nuts. It is now possible to observe a trend beginning in the form of what the body's made up of and requires and the differences in what your taste buds desire. It is important to understand how to consume food for health rather than for the pleasure of it. A typical American tastes buds are developed for acidic foods through many years of exposure to man-made food along with refined carbohydrates and tons and tons meat and other animal products. It's worth considering that the pH range of soft drinks ranges from between 2 and 2.5. This is extremely acidic, but children drink this from a lower and lower age, without hesitation. This is a real fright for taste buds that have been damaged to the point where they are actually craving things that strip paint! Acidosis can be that is caused by the over-production of acid within the blood plasma, or by an over removal of sodium bicarbonate the blood, a condition known as metabolic acidosis. It can also be caused due to the build-up of carbon dioxide in blood that result from a poor functioning of the lung or breathing problems, which is known as respiratory acidosis. When there is an increase in acid, it comes in the body, it affects the acid-base homeostasis of the body. The brain's signal triggers a breathing control system. is activated, causing more rapid and deep breathing (respiratory compensatory). The kidneys seek to compensate by creating more acid from the urine. In contrast it is possible for the body to be overwhelmed if body produces excess acid. This could lead to serious Acidosis which can lead to complications with the heart and even the coma. Acidosis is a disease that has two routes into the body, namely Respiratory and Metabolic. The metabolic acidosis is when the level of acid within the body increases due to consumption of substances that break down (metabolized) into an acid. A malfunctioning metabolism may cause metabolic acidosis. In fact, even the normal production levels of acid could result in acidosis if kidneys don't function as they should and aren't able to eliminate enough levels of acid from the urine. Acidosis in the respiratory tract occurs when lung's ability to expel carbon dioxide in a sufficient way and a condition that could occur that impacts the lungs such as pneumonia, bronchitis as well as asthma. The condition can occur in the event that brain function is impaired or muscles and nerves in the chest hinder breathing. Another way to cause respiratory acidosis occurs when breathing becomes more difficult in the body as a result of the high use of opioids (narcotics) or stronger prescription drugs to sleep (sedatives). A question I'm having is whether the prescribed drug you're using hurts or is it helping. Are you taking alkaline or acidic? If it's not derived directly from the earth nine percent of the time it's acidic. If the medication you are taking is acidic, it takes minerals away from you. Your body is forced to have to work twice as hard in order in fighting the illness, as well as the removal of minerals caused by the medication. Another thing about pH before moving to the next step. It is impossible to alter the blood's pH in the event that it does, you'd die immediately. However, various bodily fluids are affected by the rise or decrease of the pH of your blood. This is why it's a good idea for you to gradually switch into a diet that is based on plants. If it's derived from an animal, it's acidic. There's no animals that are beneficial, and there isn't any!

Electricity

Batteries are, at its core, a model of human anatomy. The battery operates using the principles of two minerals that are that are separated by a bridge of salt that permits the flow of negative and positive electrons for the creation of energy. The human body operates on electrical energy, and the brain as well as the nervous system operate on electrical. Synapsis is the brain's communication channel, which is the same as an electricity charge that is present in batteries. The greater the circulation of electrical energy in your body, the more powerful and quicker the nervous system as well as the brain are able to react. It is essential to consume foods that have a high electrical charge. What is an electrical food? They are foods that have minerals, obviously, but they must be real and natural, and preferably raw vegetables and fruits. If one eats non-mineral rich, the more energy loses and the body is affected. Like a battery that eventually gets power-depleted and so does the body. The nervous system stretches throughout the body. Every breath, reflex, idea, and action requires the use of electricity to make it happen. The nervous system acts similar to blood vessels for electricity. It is responsible for delivering the electrical pulse to targeted areas of the body is almost instantaneously. If you'd like to measure the power of your electric flow, place your toe onto one of the bedspreads. It will be easy to see and experience the speed and power of your nervous system! Within the human body, there are commonly minerals in pairs that need to exist in a particular proportion, similar to a battery in order to work properly. For instance, sodium (Na) as well as Potassium (K) are both required to be in 1 to 5 to ensure optimal health however in America the ratio is 2 to 1 which means that the majority of suffer from excessive sodium intake in their diet. A different one could be Cooper (Cu) with Zinc (Zn) which must be in an (8 (1 to) or (12 (1 to 1)) ratio to achieve optimal well-being. Copper and Zinc collaborate to enhance the immune system, nerve functions, as well as digestion. Copper as well as Zinc are in a negative relationship so if one goes not in equilibrium, one will increase. Commonly, excess zinc and copper can cause anxiety, headaches as well as depression, as well as impaired memory, just to mention several. In the United States, calcium (Ca) as well as Magnesium (Mg) in America It's a 4:1 ratio (Ca) and (Mg) However, it ought to be 1:1 percentage (Ca) (Ca) to (Mg). Calcium and Magnesium are also in synergistic relation. If either is not in balance, both will be affected. Americans consume the highest quantity of Calcium around the globe however, they suffer from the highest incidence of osteoporosis. Magnesium is required for the production of Vitamin D in the body. Vitamin D can be used to build bones, and strengthen them. The essence of it is that a deficiency of magnesium as well as excessive calcium are connected to the fractured bones that are a problem across the country. When a person is older, they're more likely suffer from mental fatigue and exhaustion which could be due to a decrease in the electrical circuits within the brain.

Chapter 2: Alkaline/Electric, TCM,
and Auryvedic Principles

The Dr. Sebi was a great source of inspiration for me and many other people. It was not my opportunity to meet him personally or even visited Usha Village in Honduras. It was fortunate for me to find the Dr. Sebi thru YouTube. After hearing his views about nutrition and health, and his personal experience, I instantly felt fascinated by him. I spent the entire night looking at videos after videos. Listening and learning from the master healer/teacher. If not the guidance of Dr. Sebi, I could not have lost over 100 pounds and changed my life for the better. One of his earliest video's, Dr. Sebi said when he was a child, he was reading a book written of Arnold Ehret that changed his life. Arnold Ehret claim to fame was the diet without mucus. The body is healed through the fasting process and eliminating excessive mucus from the body. The philosophy of his and

21

the major part of the work of Dr. Sebi was as follows. The first step was a 2-to three-day detox was recommended. If your body is leaking fluid and toxins, you should to get rid of the waste out. The best thing to do is one at least four every year. In addition, since fasting is vital to health. having regular fasting was good for your body. Self-healing of the body is a top priority. Additionally, when breaking the fast it is best to choose fruit, mostly due to their high content of water and fiber. Both of them advocated an eat-plant-based diet as the best food for humans to consume. There was a difference in the way Sebi was a doctor. Sebi taught about herbs and the benefits they could be when applied in daily life. Doctor. Sebi used his knowledge of herbal medicine to develop a variety of tonics and herbs to aid in healing the body. Numerous celebrities sought his services prior to his tragic passing in 2016.

he Traditional Chinese Medication (TCM) may be the 2nd oldest method outside of Africa with the longest-running tradition of Herbs and treatment. According to Orient mythology Li Ch'ing Yuen was said to live more than 250 years the age of his death before passing away. Chinese Modern scholars have confirmed the validity of his life. The year was 1678 when he died and he passed away in the year 1930. According to legend, he utilized TCM daily all through his life. He was also a yoga practitioner. There's a myriad of areas to be covered in the total aspects of TCM within a single section. Here is an review of this theory. All things are energy. There is no separation between the entire. Man can be an intermediary between Earth and the sky. The two are both able to transmit and receive energy through both. In TCM Ch'i, the word is to mean energy. The food we eat is energy, the air is energy and thoughts are the energy. Within the body there are energy meridians. They are referred to as the opposite energy flow Yin in and Yang. As per Taoist master Huang Keu "the Yang conserves yin and Yang radiates". An example is that of the Autonomic Nervous System, which includes two components, sympathetic and parasympathetic. Parasympathetic components are mainly targeted towards the conservation reserves, storage, and preservation of body energy. However it is the result of the sympathetic nerve stem is antagonistic as it affects the production of bodily energies as well as blocks digestion of the nutrient matter. Human body is in tandem with the nervous system autonomic. The human body is full of Ch'i that radiates into the outside world. This was not until the last few years considered a mystery, but since the advent of Kirlian photography, it has been proven that there is an aura field surrounding every living thing. Studies have revealed that the old adage of that a "green thumb" can be proven to be real. It's been established that individuals emit energy that is beneficial to the plant's aura. Conversely, a person who has"brown thumb "brown thumb" is the reverse of their energy. Within TCM there are

typically, there are five primary flavors. These also affect the main organs of the body.

Wood is a sour taste. Ch'i affects the Gall and Liver. Bladder

"Fire" = Bitter Taste The Heart is affected by Fire. Small Intestines Circulation, and Heart

Earth is sweet and has a sweet taste. Earth Ch'i affects Spleen Pancreas as well as Stomach

Metal =pungent (or spicy) flavor Metal Ch'i effects Lung and Large Intestine

Salty water flavor. influences Kidneys as well as the Bladder

In TCM the Ch'i in the body is responsible for supplying energy to twelve meridians throughout the body which herbalism is believed to have an effect on. The system is split into six parts, with each with one having a Yin quality and the other with one with a Yang quality. Each one has an elemental quality, too.

1. The Lungs are the Yin organ system that is impacted with Metal Ch'i. The lungs manage the skin, Ch'i the sinuses, larynx, pores and diaphragm.

2. The Large Intestines The Large Intestines Yang equivalent to lungs that are which are afflicted by Metal Ch'i. The large intestine functions for the removal of solid waste out of the body. It also affects the levels of water within the body as well as the quality of bodily fluids.

3. The Stomach The Stomach is a Yang organ that is influenced by the Earth Ch'i. The Ch'i in TCM is a substance extracted from the food that passes through the stomach. It is often referred to as the "Sea of Nutrition"

which is employed to facilitate extracting nutrients for your body. It is also believed to influence metabolism.

4. The Spleen The Spleen Yin organ, which is influenced by the Earth Ch'i. It influences the functions that the pancreas performs. The spleen plays a role in influencing the flow of fluid and distribution. It also is involved with Kidneys in managing the volume of fluid in the body. It helps refine and control the quality of blood.

5. The Heartis a Yin organ that is affected by fire Ch'i. Contrary to western thinking that is a part of TCM the heart regulates the activities in the cerebral cortex, as well as the limbic centre in the brain, which controls the emotion of a person. The heart controls the cardiovascular system and the circulation of blood out of the body. The function of the heart includes thyroid gland and the thymus gland and.

6. The small intestines are a Yang organ that is affected by fire Ch'i. The organ is responsible for the division of foods into organic and inorganic parts. This is the place where bacteria function plays a crucial role in nutrients absorption. It is connected to the pituitary gland that produces essential hormones needed in almost every facet of life in the organic world it is also known as the master gland.

7. The Bladder The Bladder Yang organ that is affected by water Ch'i. regulates the collection and elimination of urine. It helps balance the parasympathetic as well as sympathetic nervous systems within the body.

8. The Kidney is a Yin organ that is affected by water Ch'i. The kidney is in TCM was considered to be to be the "Root of Life". The kidneys filter blood and eliminate the cellular waste, and also excess water and also. The kidneys control the relationship between acid and base of body fluids within

the body via a sequence of chemical reactions involving minerals such as sodium, potassium ammonia, bicarbonate and ammonia. The kidneys contain adrenal glands too they control the creation of steroids and hormones in the body. The kidneys are also responsible for controlling hair that grows on the head as well as facial and pubic hair.

9. It is the Gall Bladder- Yang organ is affected through Wood Ch'i. regulates the flow of Bile throughout the body. It is essential for the digestion of oily and fat-rich meals.

10. Circulation-Sexis usually linked to the pericardium the heart's protective shell is can be described as a Yin the fire-system. It is a term used in the west that is comparable with the spiritual. It influences the feelings of love, which is displayed sexually, as a link between emotions and sexual intimacy.

11. The Triple Warmer, Yang and Fire is that is connected with the hypothalamus which is a brain part that is responsible for a variety of bodily functions such as the creation of hormones as well as appetite and temperature control and more.

12. The Liveris the Yin organ that is affected by Wood Ch'i. The liver is the place where blood flows in our body in order to detoxify. The liver is home to a huge part of sugar in form of Glycogen and is ready to enter the bloodstream to perform work. The majority of the hormones and proteins that are present in our body are broken down by the liver. It is the peripheral nerve system (nerves that originate out of the central nerve system) is linked to the liver via TCM that is directly linked with the eye and the body, as well. As a result of sexual intimacy, the Liver is believed to provide vitality to the sexual organs.

Ayurveda has been practiced for over 7000 years, and was first developed by Indians as well as Hindus. Ayurveda is a variety of research. The most popular branch is Rasayana. Rasmeans primordial tissue, or plasma, and ayana means pathway. The word itself refers to the path taken by plasma. Within the various branches of research, Rasayana is the area that is associated with rejuvenation of the body. In Ayurveda the duration of humans is divided into 4 distinct phases.

1.) From birth to around 20 years of age the body's tissues are developing.

2.) Between 20-40 years old, with tissues that are remain growing

3.) between 40 and 60, the time of plateau. In addition, if one is eating well, has a good mental health, and is free from stress and worry This stage could be utilized to increase capacity for mental toughness.

4.) After 60, no matter how good of life, certain activities decrease. For instance, metabolism, bone and tendon loss as cognitive decline.

In the stages 3 and 4, this is where Rasayana proved to be particularly effective in regenerating the body. Like TCM studies, the purpose behind Rasayana helps to improve the balance in the body with the use of different rasas (associated with a distinct taste). Everything we eat is a combination of one or more the six rasas.

1.) Sweet ras, primarily is found in carbs like starch and sugar-rich products. It provides energy to bones, semen blood, liver, and flesh. When it is in excess, it can lead to laziness hypertension, diabetes as well as weight gain.

2.) Acidic rasis commonly connected with acidic fruit as well as fermented food. It affects saliva and improves digestion. It can also acidify the body.

3.) Salty ras, which is found in minerals, it makes foods more appealing. The excess of salt may cause appetite, loss of hair as well as a decrease in sexual energy.

4.) Bitter ras- the main comprised of herbs. It alkalizes the body, eliminates cell waste and strengthens and strengthens the body. When it is used in excess, it can act as an anti-inflammatory agent.

5.) RAS-Pungent Spices that are utilized to provide the food flavor and zest. They help eliminate microbes that are present in the food. In excess, it can cause sedation or insanity.

6.) Astringent ras- typically found in unripe fruits, the roots and barks. If it is excessive, it can be detrimental on the nervous system.

In addition to the six Ras, there are three different doshas. Vata, Pitta, and Kapha which are similar to air, bile and the phlegm. They are synergistic with various ras and they are affected in a different way by the other. Vata is reduced by sweet ras, sharp and sweet ras lowers pitta and so on.

Vata is the vital force of our body, which is a part of the air. It is responsible for separating cells into various types, forms blood vessels, nerves and other structures. If vata functions properly, the senses of all five are healthy, even if it is, then death or illness could take place.

Pitta creates and keeps the body warmth that's in conjunction with the bile. The Pitta enzyme is involved to aid digestion, metabolic function and in nutrient absorption. In close contact with the spleen and liver for the production of blood. In excess of hot, spicy, fried and salty foods can trigger the pitta gland to overflow. In excess pitta, it can cause an increase in calcium levels acidity, headaches or.

Kapha that is associated with phlegm offers cooling properties and is a good condition for mucous membranes, bile and the gastric juices. Kapha is afflicted by acidic, sweet and hard-to digest foods. This causes the common cold asthma, and cough flare-ups. It increases saliva and mucus production.

Chapter 3: The Profit of Disease

The amount of people who used at least one prescription medication within the past 30 days. This includes women and men of any race. 1988-1994 =39.1%, 1999-2002=45.2%, 2007-2010=47.5% and 2011-2014= 47.0%

The percentage of patients who have taken three or more prescription medications over the past 30 days, including males and females and races. 1988-1994=11.8%, 1999-2002=17.8%, 2007-2010=20.8% and 2011-2014=21.5%

The percentage of patients who have taken 5 or more prescription medications over the past 30 days, including males and females and race. 1988-1994=4.0%, 1999-2002=7.5%, 2007-2010=10.1% and 2011-2014=10.9%

It's clear that the amount of people taking prescription drugs has been on increasing in a steady manner for nearly twenty years.

The estimates suggest that 70 % of the American populace is using at least one prescription medication regularly.

Here's a complete The list of pharmaceutical company's revenue for 2015 and 2016.

1.) Johnson and Johnson; 70.04 billion and 71.89 billion

2.) Pfizer; 48.85 billion and 52.82 billion

3.) Roche; 47.70 billion and 50.11 billion

4.) Novartis; 49.41 billion and 48.52 billion

5.) Merck; 29.5 billion and 39.8 billion

6.) Sanofi; 36.73 billion and 36.57 billion

7.) GlaxoSmithKline; 29.84 billion and 34.79 billion

8.) Gilead Sciences; 32.15 billion and 30.39 billion

9) AbbVie 22.82 billion, and 25.56 billion

10.) Bayer; 24.09 billion and 25.27 billion

These 10 companies made more than 300 billion dollars each year. It is now clear the profits behind Big Pharmaceutical. Drug companies employ drug representatives who travel from doctor offices to physicians' offices to promote their employers' products. Reps from drug companies even visit the pharmacy to sell their product. Did you know that doctors receive rewards from pharmaceutical companies when prescribing one drug over other, not simply because one is better, but simply due to the fact that doctors will earn a fee for every patient who take that specific medication? In the wake of Obama's Obama legislation on healthcare, drug manufacturers are now required to disclose the public information about their payments to doctors. Analysts are required to comply with the law. They have developed the program Open Payments, where patients are able to determine if there is there is a conflict of interests in the event of a medicine or. A pharmaceutical company has was able to spend more than $36,000,000 on general payment and $45 million for research-related payments. The company also stated "Compensation for other services that consulting services, such as being a faculty member or speakers at events that is not an ongoing education program". This same pharmaceutical firm in that year also paid two doctors more than $600,000 to prescribe specific prescriptions. That's not to suggest physicians aren't trying to earn extra cash. However, the big pharmaceutical companies are essentially battling in the field of medicine. According to estimates going to the past 20 years that at least 100,000 individuals die every year from adverse reactions caused by prescription medicines. A 1998 article from the American Medical Association projected 106,000 deaths in that one year. Based on the most recent forecasts, are concerned, the figure is higher than 125,000 per year. Prof. Donald Light at the Rowan University of Osteopathic Medicine claims that "about two-thirds of people a week will be killed by drugs appropriately prescribed. This is according to detailed charts of patients admitted to hospitals".

The need for treatment and the number that is harmful are two fundamental concepts the majority of people haven't heard previously. Every drug on the market must be evaluated to determine its quality and safety. Once the tests are completed and the results are returned the number needed for treatment is provided. It means that for every one individual who is benefited by the drug, a specific amount of patients either do not experience any result or experience a side-effect of the drug. One example is one of the most low-dose Aspirin (acetaminophen) which is believed to lower the likelihood of suffering a heart attack. Take a look at the numbers that needs to be treated, which is 1 per year for 1667. It means that in every 1667 individuals who take aspirin at a low dose daily for a year, just one will be able to avoid a heart problem. The amount of treatment required the risk of the risk of a heart attack that is not life-threatening is one in 2000 over one year. To prevent Strokes and heart attacks, a low dose of Aspirin is advised to be taken. The amount needed for treatment is one in three for one year. For every 3000 individuals who take this medicine, only one person is protected from strokes that are not life-threatening.

The amount of harm that is needed is the opposite of the amount needed to treat. This is the amount of individuals who are taking a specific prescription, over time that are exposed to negative effects that resulted in harm to one individual but not the other. If you are taking the low dosage Aspirin the required number of people to cause harm is one per 3333 over the course of a year. For every 3333 individuals who took the low dose of aspirin over a year, one victim was "harmed" and when it comes to

the low dose of aspirin, was an extremely
bleeding event.

Chapter 4: Thyroid

The thyroid medication is among the most commonly prescribed medicines in America. It is consistently among the top three prescribed medications every year. There are many people who suffer from thyroid issues, and some require having the thyroid gland removed by surgery. What exactly is the functions of the thyroid gland as well as its importance in our bodies? The thyroid gland is a part of the endocrine system in your body. The endocrine systems are similar with the nerve system both of which are main systems within the human body. They manage and control the various body system. The endocrine gland produces and distributes chemical messengers known as hormones to the body. The hormones function as switches on and off within cells. It informs the cells that they must perform the job they are supposed to do or to stop performing a specific task. The glands have various functions within the body, such as the thalamus gland pituitary gland, pineal gland, adrenal glands tests and ovaries. They each produce different hormones. The thyroid gland is located in the neck, ahead of the larynx, thyroid gland makes two primary hormones, namely triiodothyronine and thyrox. Thyroxine's primary function is to trigger the metabolism of Oxygen which fuels metabolism in the tissues and cells of the body. Thyroxine is known as T4 and triiodothyronine called T3. Thyroxine (T4) is the messenger hormone in the thyroid gland. It is produced by the thyroid gland, and then flows into the bloodstream, transferring to targeted cells. There, it's transformed into T3. After being converted into triiodothyronine it transforms into the active version of thyroid hormone. This starts metabolism. It is the method by which food is broken down into smaller molecules so that are absorbed by the body. The mechanism for thyroid hormones within the cell functions to connect to the nucleus as well as cell receptors, and then copy DNA to produce proteins. It is controlled by the pituitary gland, which is responsible for the production of thyroid stimulant hormone (TSH). The pituitary gland in the brain gets data from the body using indicators like metabolic rate, blood pressure, and various other signals. It reacts by either growing TSH production, which is then transferred into the thyroid gland, increasing the production of thyroxine, or reducing TSH production, which reduces the production of Thyroxine. When diagnosing thyroid disorders, TSH levels are checked throughout the body. The presence of low levels of TSH detected in the body is known as hypothyroidism. While high levels of TSH that are found within the body is referred to as hyperthyroidism. A low level of TSH is typically treated by "synthetic TSH" in a tablet format. In contrast, high levels TSH are treated by radioactive iodine, which lowers the level.

Let's look at the hormone made in the thyroid gland. In order for Thyroxine (T4) to make it, the body requires 4 Iodine-containing atoms in order to bond with the amino acid. The reason Iodine is so important and its significance important is that the body is unable to make the mineral. Iodine needs to be consumed by eating food items to make it into the body. If it isn't absorbed each day through the food that we consume, the thyroid gland will not be in a position to produce this crucial hormone and its substitute, triiodothyronine (T3).

Here are some indications that are indicative of Hypothyroidism (low the amount of Iodine)

1) Hair loss

2.) Skin and hair that are dry.

3) Fatigue

4.) The weight gain or the difficulty of in losing weight due to a reduced calorific consumption

5) Aches and muscle cramps

6) Decreased Libido

7) Menstrual cycle irregularity

8) Constipation

9) Depression

10) The sensitivity to cold

Synthetic T4 replacements consist of a sodium salt tetraiodothyronine made of synthetic conception but is identical to the hormone produced from the Thyroid gland. A few of the "inactive" substances are magnesium stearate confectioner's sugar (which includes corn starch) for a mere handful of. It is interesting to note the color additives utilized for color, such as Red No. 40 Aluminum Lake and Yellow No.6 Aluminum Lake. Red 40 is a color addition that can be found in many of items. It is derived from petroleum distillates and coal Tars. According to the Center for Sciences in the Public Interest says "Red 40 and various other colors can trigger allergies in certain people". Research has shown that they can cause the hyperactivity of children, as well as cancers of the immune system in rodents. One of the ingredients that is present in Red 40 is p-Cresidine, that is "reasonably expected" as a carcinogen according to the Department of Human Health Services. If you are taking synthetic thyroid, dosages and concentrations must be controlled. If they are not, there could be consequences upon development and growth and bone metabolism, digestive processes, reproduction function mood and the metabolism of lipids and glucose.

Women, thyroid replacement has been proven to boost bone resorption and consequently reducing bone mineral density for women postmenopausal taking higher doses of replacement as well as in women taking doses that suppress the effects that contain synthetic thyroid. The increase in bone resorption could be due to an increase in urine excretion of calcium and

Phosphorus, in addition to the suppression of levels of parathyroid hormone.

When taking synthetic hormones it is important to know that there are additional drugs used in combination with them that may create an Drug interaction. Drug interaction. The drugs can reduce the absorption of T4 which can cause hypothyroidism.

Antacids (Aluminum and Magnesium)

Ferrous Sulfate

Calcium Carbonate

Hydroxides (Simethicone)

Iodine is an elemental mineral which can't be made in the human body. It is ingested through the food we eat or through other supplements. The thyroid requires minimum 70 mg of Iodine in order to make the hormone thyroxine (T4) along with triiodothyronine (T3). Iodine is essential for kids because it aids in the mental and physical growth. Iodine in sufficient amounts helps in the development of the fundamental abilities including language, movement and hearing. Iodine is essential for overall IQ. A typical adult requires about 150 micrograms per daily. Children aged 12 months and younger require around 120 micrograms per every day. Kids aged 8 to 12 years old require around 80 micrograms. For children aged 13 years old, the recommended quantity is around 130 milligrams. Mothers who are expecting and breastfeeding require 220 and 290 micrograms per daily, and 290 micrograms, respectively. Adults, the recommended quantity for the maximum amount of intake is 1,000 micrograms daily.

Electric/Alkaline thyroid herb Bladderwrack (Fucus vesiculosus) contains the highest amount of Iodine in the natural world. Bladderwrack is composed of iodine and calcium as well as magnesium as well as sodium, potassium iron, silicon, B complex vitamin minerals and trace metals the phenolics and lipids, as well as algin and the phlorotannins. The other constituents include Vitamin A, C,E, K,S, and G. The use of Bladderwrack was for centuries to treat thyroid problems. A bottle of Bladderwrack supplements may be as high as 600 micrograms for each gram of Iodine that is naturally occurring.

TCM medicine to treat thyroid

Panax Ginseng one of the most popular herbal remedies that of all time is commonly utilized. It is a component of TCM where thyroid glands being a component in the body's endocrine systems, as well in connection with pituitary glands, a Yang Herb is best suited. Panax Ginseng is believed to help replenish and replace the loss of Ch'i within the organs and energy meridians. Panax Ginseng is a product of China, Japan, or Korea. The term Panax comes from the Greek term "panacea" meaning "cure all' or "remedy to cure all diseases'. Panax Ginseng is taste that is sweet, but slightly bitter. The main ingredient in the Panax Ginseng is Panaquilon which acts as an endocrine stimulant and regulates the endocrine system. Most likely to be found in the hypothalamus and pituitary glands that produce TSH.

The herb Ayurveda/Rasayana for thyroid is used in conjunction

Ashwagandha (Withania somnifera)is also referred to by the name of Indian Ginseng shows very promising results on thyroid. The range of effects varies from Auryvedic to sweet RAS and a disturbance in Pitta is linked with an imbalance in the thyroid gland. Studies on mice showed that they were treated with ashwagandha. Then, the thyroid hormone levels were measured. The treatment increased T3 levels by 18%, and T4 levels up to 111% in just 20 days. The human study participants receiving Ashwagandha showed an increase in TSH along with increased T4 levels from the beginning to all the way to 24 percentage.

Guggul (Commiphora Mukul). According to research, Guggul helps fight against the thyroid gland's inefficiency by increasing the conversion rate of T4 into T3 that is the most potent type of the thyroid hormone. Around 80% of T4 as well as 20% are produced in the gland of thyroid. The majority of T3 is created in extracellular tissues through the conversion of T4 into T3. T3 has around 4 times as much hormone power that T4 has.

Dietary supplements for thyroid

Kelp, Dulse, Nori, Wakame and Sea moss are a few examples of sea-based vegetables. The cranberries are an excellent source too. Around four ounces of cranberries have 400 micrograms of iodine. It is preferring organic when is possible. A medium sized organic potato that has the skin on is about 60 micrograms iodine.

Chapter 5: Hypertension

Prior to the 1900's, the high blood pressure didn't exist as an identifiable "disease". The sphygmometer wasn't (a device to measure blood pressure) created until the early 1900's. Everyone knew about the symptoms that are associated with Hypertension and the best way to manage it. A few of the signs were: Obesity, Diabetes, Erectile Dysfunction, Kidney Disease and heart diseases to name just a handful. What exactly is blood pressure determined?

A Sphygmometer

BP class Systolic Diastolic

mm Hg (upper#) mm Hg (lower #)

Normal less than 120, and less than 120

Prehypertension 120-139 or 80-89

High BP and the stage 1 hypertension 140-150, or 90-100

High BP High BP, Stage 2 hypertension of 160 or more or 100 or more

Hypertensive Crises 180 or more or 110 or more

The blood pressure inside the body changes constantly. The body can be tested ten times time intervals and receive different results. The general rule is to take a test every 2 or 3 days during the day for a week, and then take the mean of the tests approximately. A different indicator for hypertension would be the rates of heart. Normal heart rate ranges from 60 to 100 beats per minute. The 70-80 range is considered to be normal. Any beat that is higher than 80 Beats Per Minute is typically an indication of high blood pressure.

As the heart beats, it increases the pressure of the arteries and equals Systolic tension (upper #) during beats. The pressure within the arteries reduces, which is equal to diastolic pressure (lower #)

The heart contains four chambers.

Right atrium that draws blood from veins, and then pumps it to the right ventricle.

The right ventricle absorbs the blood pumped by the right atrium. It then transports it to the lungs. There, it's oxygenated.

Left atrium It is where oxygenated blood comes from the lungs. It then pump it to the left ventricle.

The left ventricle (the largest chamber) circulates oxygenated blood throughout other parts of our body. Its intense contractions generate blood pressure.

There are coronary veins that can be found on the exterior of the heart, which provide oxygenated blood flow to the muscle of the heart. The web-like network of nerve tissues is found throughout the heart and transmits signals which control contracture and relaxation. The heart's surround is a sac known as the pericardium. This in TCM is connected to the Circulation-sex Meridian.

Primary hypertension causes up to 85 percent of hypertension that is diagnosed, commonly referred to as the lifestyle disorder. The causes of these are typically issues that can be addressed with no drugs, and usually without herbal remedies, but only with changes in lifestyle and diet. Secondary hypertension generally occurs with people who are younger. In most cases, the hormonal system and birth defects can be the cause to secondary hypertension.

Causes of High Blood Pressure

The blood pressure rises with older age. Blood vessels become less elastic as we get older. This can lead to atherosclerosis.

Potassium and Vitamin D insufficiency

High Salt (Sodium) intake

People with excess weight tend to be more likely to develop of HBP

Variation in Hormones may impact BP levels

If Kidneys function isn't working properly, could cause HBP

Anxiety and Stress could trigger an increase in BP

Genetics may be a determining factor

Race (African American) are more at chance to develop Hypertension

Diabetics are more likely to experience instances of HBP

The risk of smoking cigarettes is higher be suffering from HBP than non-smokers.

The general diagnosis of any four of these are often utilized to determine hypertension.

1) Shortness of Breath

2) Dizziness

3) Heartbeats are increased or palpated. beats

4) Trembling

5) Sweating

6) Nausea, stomach upset or vomiting

7) Numbness, tingling

8.) Flashes of cold or hot

9) Chest pains

10.) Afraid of losing your life, or the fear of becoming insane

HBP- The Silent Killer

Hypertension is thought to be one of the main or major reason for the death of more than 1000 people every day across the United States.

HBP is the primary reason for stroke.

HBP is the main trigger for Heart attack

6.9% those who've experienced their first heart attack. 77% of those with had their first stroke. 74% of those with heart failure also suffer from HBP.

"In the United States, 1 out 3 (31 percent) of the population that is adult suffers from elevated blood pressure. It's a minimum of 80 million people. Of these, just half can control their blood pressure.

A further 30 percent of people have prehypertension

The most common treatment of HBP is:

1.) Diuretics- enhance the kidneys' mechanism of action by encouraging the excretion of excess water. Utilizing diuretics for long periods of time for managing HBP greatly depletes your body of vital minerals. The minerals that are excreted through the fluids of inside the body are magnesium sodium, potassium as well as zinc and iodine. Diuretics hinder the kidney's capacity to absorb these minerals, particularly sodium.

2.) Alpha-adrenergic blockers as well as Beta blockers. Alpha and Beta blockers are designed to weaken the heart and ease the blood vessels. Beta blockers eliminate the capacity of the heart to adrenaline and epinephrine that stimulates the heart's pulse of the heart as well as blood pressure rises, thereby increasing both. In their design, the drugs are intended be used to "weaken" the cardiovascular system, so that blood pressure can be reduced, and heart discomfort is reduced.

3.) Calcium channel blockers, Ace inhibitors and angiotensin II receptor blocking agents lower blood pressure through stopping the flow of Calcium to those arterial walls cells. This causes blood vessels to relax and less constricted. Calcium is required in the body to perform a range of functions in the cardiovascular system, including contraction mechanisms of the heart as well as the smooth muscle. Additionally, it is required to store and release energy within cells. The use of calcium blockers is not recommended for a long time. Any medication that interferes with your body's normal function and hinders the usage of this vital mineral will not be helpful for the long haul.

A lot of times, multiple kinds of medications are prescribed in conjunction with each other for the treatment of HBP.

Common Adverse Reaction to Antihypertensive Diuretics

Menstrual Inconsistency

Sexual dysfunction

Gastrointestinal problems

Nausea

Glucose intolerance

Hypokalemia

Hypercholesterolemia

Gynecomastia

Common Adverse Reaction of Alpha and Beta Blockers

Sexual dysfunction

Insomnia

Fatigue

Less HDL cholesterol

Bronchospasm

Increases the risk of heart failure

Masking hyperglycemia

Commonly occurring adverse reactions of Calcium channel blockers ACE inhibitors as well as Angiotensin II receptor blockers

Rash

Sexual dysfunction

Angioedema

Headache

Hyperkalemia

The number needed to be treated patients who have mild hypertension but no cardiovascular condition that was not present before they used blood pressure medications for five years in order to stop the death of a cardiovascular patient and strokes: 1 out of 1 for the likelihood of total death

1 out of 82 are at risk for heart death

1 out of 172 is a stroke

The number required to the harm caused by people who were taking antihypertensive medicines for five years, the following was reported:

1 out of 10 patients were harmed (experienced negative side effects and stopped treatment).

Hypertension isn't a singular condition, but is a manifestation of numerous other issues that remain not readily apparent. This is why Hypertension is referred to by the name of "silent death knell". Treatment for hypertension in the conventional way involves lowering and maintaining control over blood pressure through "lessening" the power in the cardiovascular system, its absorption and utilization of minerals, as well as to block the body's own natural mechanisms. According to TCM there are a variety of causes for Hypertension include:

1) Constitution -

2.) Overextended Yang Hyper-achiever, Go-getter. Expels a lot of Yang (heat)

3.) Insufficient YinPeople with excessive Yang suffer from lower Yin (cool) energetic energy inside their bodies. Yang is like the motor of cars, and Yin is similar to the oil in the motor.

4.) Diet- You are the food you consume

5) Insufficient exercise

6.) Lack of rest Melatonin which is the "sleep hormone" could

7) Stress

TCM herbs for hypertension

Hibiscus (Hibiscus Sabdariffa) that is utilized in TCM as well as Auryvedic practices it is highly potent anti-hypertensive herbal. It is often compared with ACE inhibitors such as Lisinopril or Captopril. Hibiscus is diuretic, it is less in blood, the less pressure. Additionally, by functioning as an ACE inhibitor, it eases tension in the capillary and small arteries systems in the heart (Nwachukwu DC in 2015). Around 1/3 of blood flow is contained in blood vessels, and easing tension will decrease blood pressure. Based on research, 2-3 cups per daily of hibiscus tea are required for therapeutic dosage. A study showed that hibiscus tea to be equally effective, if it is not more effective in treating mild to moderate hypertension as hydrochlorothiazide (HCTZ). Contrary to HCTZ that can alter the electrolyte balance within our bodies, hibiscus didn't.

Eucommia bark/Tu Chung (Eucommia Ulmoides) is a kidney Yang tonic that is that is used to treat kidneys as well as liver meridians within the body. Through clinical studies, Eucommia bark was found to contain blood pressure-lowering components that act as the natural beta-adrenergic antagonist to assist in dilation of blood vessels (Greenway F, 2011,). Eucommia has been proven to contain a high amount of amino acids as well as minerals, vitamins as well as flavonoids. Flavonoids are chemicals that are naturally occurring and are regarded as secondary metabolites that are used as chemical messengers. They also play a role in regulation of body functions and inhibitors of cell cycle. Seven various flavonoids were isolated from the eucommia. What's great about this plant is that it has no interaction with drugs. There are no known side effects.

Hawthorne fruits (Crataegus) can also be employed in treating hypertension. Hawthorne helps to increase blood flow in smaller vessels. Hawthorne serves as an naturally ACE inhibitor, calcium blocker, as well as Nitric Oxide release (vasodilator) to lower blood pressure, and stop the production of angiotensin, which is a blood vessel dilator that is responsible for raising blood pressure. Hawthorne can be a food source for elderly heart, hypertensive and myocardial insufficiency or cardiac arrhythmias and angina. It is not recommended for pregnant women, or for those using Warfarin (may cause an increase in anticoagulation).

It is believed that Ayurveda (Rasayana) Hypertension can be defined in the form of Rakta Gata Vata. Rakta Gata Vata is essentially an affliction of blood triggered by excessive pitta and vata. Kapha is also compromised, resulting in loss and assistance for the cardiovascular system. The Ayurveda vata which is situated within the colon. Toxins within the colon may be taken up into blood, causing constrictions to blood vessels, particularly the arterial. Vata inside the colon is dry and cold, which eventually results in constipation. Vata hypertension can increase due to emotional stress, anxiety and general anxiety. The small intestines found in Ayurveda is where the body stores pittas in our bodies. Food-borne toxins derived from undigested foods are found in the intestines circulate throughout the body. The toxins trigger the blood to become viscous. The increase in viscosity triggers the blood to put pressure on blood vessels. When pitta is present, hypertension can increase due to strong emotions, such as fear, anger or jealousy. Kapha is located within the stomach. According to Ayurveda, Kapha like gastric secretions participate in digesting of carbohydrates, starch and glucose. The result of this process of digestion is the triglycerides. If Kapha in the stomach gets disrupted, there's an increase in the triglycerides level and cholesterol (which is an alternative variant of the kapha). The blood thickens and cause fatty particles to accumulate in blood vessels. This can lead to a narrowing of the blood vessels and the possibility of a heart attack. The hypertension that occurs in Kapha may be caused by dysfunction of vital organs in the body (liver kidney, heart as well as the kidneys).

Ayurveda/Rasayana herbs for hypertension

Ashwagandha (Withania somnifera) often referred to in the form of Indian Ginseng has been used in Ayurveda from the beginning of time. Ashwagandha is utilized in the body to alleviate stress through its moderate effect on the body's sedative. Its anti-stress qualities are the reason it's employed to treat hypertension. It has been proven to reverse adrenal depletion caused by stress. Ashwagandha is an natural calcium channel blocking agent and as a beta blocker. It has the ability to lower blood pressure systolic. Calcium dilates the heart. excess calcium is present in our body, which keeps the heart contracting and at ease.

Arjuna (Terminalia arjuna) is an Ayurveda herb that is used to treat hypertension too. Arjuna bark contains organic antioxidants (flavonoids) and saponins. coenzyme Q-10, as well as minerals such as zinc, magnesium copper, magnesium, as well as calcium. Co-enzyme Q-10 is one of the vital molecule for ATP and is the energy source for every cell. It is possible for the body to make co-enzyme 10, but the production begins slowing around 50 years of age. Heart muscle cells need lots of metabolic energy in order to function, specifically as they're always in operation. The benefits that coenzyme Q10 are numerous. It has the ability to enhance energy production, serve as an antioxidant and help stabilize membrane fluidity, thus reducing blood viscosity, and decreasing the risk of hypertension. If you are suffering with cardiovascular issues or simply need to ensure that your heart's function within a normal range You may want to supplement your diet with coenzymeQ10. Coenzyme Q10 10 is beneficial to cardiovascular health and has been proven to reduce the risk of heart attacks. Arjuna works as the body's natural beta blocker the body. It was scientifically tested to increase the systolic blood pressure within the body. The herb has diuretic qualities that are mild, reduce blood lipid levels and aid in reducing the formation of blood clots.

Tulsior Holy Basil (Ocimum Sanctum) is among the main herbs that are used in Ayurvedic practice. It is often referred to as "The The Queen of herbs" or the "Elixir of Life". It is used to neutralize kapha as well as to regulate vata and pitta throughout the body. Holy Basil is considered an adaptogen. It is a plant that improves the body's reaction to tension. Tannings, flavonoids, vital oils, calcium the iron chlorophyll manganese, sodium and Vitamins A and C can be present inside Holy Basil. It is a great source of Magnesium that relaxes the heart Holy basil is proven to lower blood pressure effect. A study conducted on animals, holy basil reduced the systolic blood pressure to 20 mmHg, and also decreased diastolic blood pressure to 15 millimeters over a four-week duration.

The Winter Melon (Ash Gourd) is utilized as part of the Ayurvedic method of healing and is used for its medicinal properties. It is classified as a vegetable but not as a fruit, it's only plant in the Benincasa hispida Genus. There are some constituents that have a high content of Vitamin C as well as B2 iron, zinc, potassium and phosphorous as well as calcium as well as niacin, thiamine, as well as some amino acids. The rind is known to contain diuretic qualities, which aids the body in eliminate toxins and reduce blood pressure. Due to its rich content of Potassium and Vitamin C, winter melon has proven to be highly effective for maintaining cardiovascular health. Potassium is vasodilator. This means it reduces blood pressure by release of tension that's build up in blood vessels and the arteries, which allows blood flow to flow more easily.

Electric/Alkaline Herbs

Cayenne Pepper (Capsicum Annum) is included on the Doctor. Sebi nutritional guide list as an alternative for alkaline-based seasoning. Cayenne Pepper is known to have an effect that moves blood in your body that causes a warmth when it is digested. Cayenne pepper contains Vitamin A, Vitamin B6, Vitamin E, Vitamin C, Vitamin B2, manganese and potassium. One of the Cayenne Pepper's main ingredient is capsaicin. This has been proven to lower blood pressure throughout the body.

Cayenne Pepper has been proven to be a the natural ACE inhibition effect in relation to blood pressure.

Valerian The Valerian (Valeriana officinalis) is used for an sedative as well as a sleep aid. It assists in relaxing your body and fights anxiety. It reduces stress within the body, and due to its sedative properties It has also been proven to decrease blood pressure and. Valerian root consists of iron, calcium, manganese and magnesium zinc, selenium, Vitamin B Vitamins, Vitamin C and essential acid fatty acids. Additionally, it is a source of phytonutrients, such as BetaCarotene, also known as Beta Carotene which is an excellent antioxidant powerhouse that is great for heart health, as well as Limonene that falls within the classification of Terpenes. Limonene can be found in the oils of citrus peels. It has been proven that limonene may trigger anapoptosis (death signal) that kills cancer cells and stops cancerous cells from reproducing. Limonene increases the amount of liver enzymes which help to eliminate carcinogens within the body.

Soursop (Guanabana) is an indigenous fruit from South America. Soursop is rich in amino acids Vitamin B, Vitamin C folate, iron Vitamin E, Vitamin k as well as potassium, selenium as well as zinc. The leaves of the tree are also a source of Co Q-10, which has been proven to reduce both diastolic and systolic blood pressures in humans. Studies on animals showed that Soursop worked in the role of an vasodilator (relaxes tension in the arteries and blood vessels) and also has an antihypertensive (low blood pressure) qualities. Potassium levels that are high that are present in Soursop is extremely beneficial. potassium reduces the negative effects of sodium on the body.

Certain foods can help reduce blood pressure

The extract of olive leaf is an excellent natural remedy to treat hypertension. The extract of olive leaves contains triterpenes and flavonoids. One of the most important phytonutrients that Oleuropein contains is known as a Polyphenol. Oleuropein is a potent antioxidant. It has been proven to function as an natural vasodilator, allowing improved blood flow and because it is an effective antioxidant, it can get rid of harmful free radicals within the body. Free radicals are known to trigger inflammation of blood vessels and arteries, which in turn LDL cholesterol could connect to inflamed regions. This could cause blood vessels and arteries to shrink and increase blood pressure. Olive leaf is proven and found to be just as effective as Captopril the drug used in pharmaceuticals, which is an artificial ACE inhibitor.

Watercress (Nasturtium Officinale) is a leafy, green leafy vegetable, that grows naturally from spring water. It has been proven by research that watercress has the highest concentration of nutrients-rich vegetable on the planet. It is a rich source of Vitamins A, C, B1,B1, B6, E,K, calcium, folic acid manganese, iodine Zinc, phosphorous magnesium and phytonutrients such as beta-carotene as well as quercetin, glucosinolate and beta-caro. The nutrient known as lutein that's healthy for eyes, has proven to lower blood pressure through reducing the thickness of the arterial wall, which can lead to inadequate circulation. A cup of watercress contains more than 100% daily requirement of Vitamin K in its own. Due to its rich mineral content particularly magnesium and calcium, and magnesium, which play a synergistic roles in the regulation of blood pressure, it is a plant that must be included in every eating plan.

Chapter 6: Diabetes In order to learn more about

Diabetes and what it is, it's important to look from the Pancreas. In the endocrine system pancreas organ is located in the abdominal area within the body. It is situated in the stomach behind and connects to the small intestinal tract. It plays two important duties in the body. foremost, it assists in digestion. Once food is at the tip in the intestines of small size the pancreas releases an acid that is laden with enzymes which begin breaking down the food. Additionally, the pancreas aids in control blood sugar levels throughout the body, by releasing hormones. Blood sugar (sugar) levels need to be kept at a certain level throughout the body. The body needs to maintain a continuous flow of sugar in order to nourish cells, but not so excessively that kidneys as well as other organs get adversely affected. The pancreas makes two hormones that help to maintain blood sugar level: Glucagon is a hormone that increases sugar levels through activating the liver to convert sugar into glucose molecules that can be released into blood. The second hormone is Insulin which decreases blood glucose levels following eating by triggering the absorption of glucose the liver, the muscles and fat tissues.

The term "diabetes" is used to refer to either diabetic mellitus or diabetes. If you are talking about the term diabetes, most people refer the condition known as diabetes mellitus. Diabetes insipidus is a very rare uncomplicated disorder. It is divided into two types Type 1 (insulin dependent) and type 2 (non-insulin dependent).

We will look at the way that insulin can play a part within the body.

Food can be divided into three distinct categories: proteins, fats and carbohydrates. Three carbs, carbohydrates increase blood sugar levels within the body at the fastest rate. Carbohydrates consist of sugar starch. When you consume carbohydrates, especially ones with low fiber content and insulin is released, it can transport glucose to cells. The cells are equipped with insulin receptors connected to them, which permit cells to take in sugar and produce energy. The process of metabolism will only occur at a specific rate, so the extra glucose needs to be stored elsewhere within the body. It is stored in glycogen that is stored in the body, it can store up to 200 grams glucose within the muscles, as well as 70 grams of glucose within the liver. If those two areas have been filled, insulin receptors are reduced on those cells, so that glucose doesn't get into. The extra glucose must be moved somewhere, and one of the worst locations is the bloodstream. Once glucose is introduced into the bloodstream, it begins to connect to proteins via an process known as Glycation. Glycation occurs when glucose in bloodstreams attaches with proteins, lipids and nucleic acid, and results in Advanced Glycation End-Products (AGE). A good example from Nature could be the maturing process that occurs in an apple. After the course of time it is common for dark spots to develop on a banana that's sweet. The similar thing occurs in our body when there is age. These are referred to as glycotoxins and when present in large quantities in the body could cause hypertension, diabetes as well as other chronic illnesses. The difficulty with having too many AGE's that are present in our bodies, particularly for diabetics is their ability to be absorbed into capillaries and bloodstream. The majority of diabetics suffer from blindness or even have a foot, leg or toe cut off because of these areas with very tiny arteries in which it is easy for glycotoxins to accumulate and cause harm.

After the body has stored all of the glucose it needs in its organs and the liver, and does not want to allow the excessive Glycation process to take place, it lowers the insulin receptors found on a majority of cells and prevents glucose from getting enter. The glucose that is left over breaks into the triglycerides that are stored in the one area where insulin cell receptors actually are growing, and that's in the fat cells in the body! Anywhere there's insulin, there is fat and both of them are connected. In order to utilize the energy stored within the fat tissue the fatty acids are taken from the tissues and broken down into energy, thereby causing you to lose the fat. When insulin levels are excessive, it is impossible to reduce the fat tissue. The enzyme which allows fat acids to break down from fat storage is called Hormone Sensitive Lipidase that's insulin-sensitive and won't allow fat to break it down in the presence of insulin. If there's excessive insulin levels in the body, you are unable to use stored fat and it is always difficult to eat and fatigued. The only energy source your body is able to burn is glucose. This causes the body to consume more and more, to replenish your energy. This causes you to gain weight.

Sucrose (table sugar) is comprised of one portion fructose and one portion glucose. Sucrose can be found in more than 80percent of the items at the supermarket. It is referred to as diabetes because it contains sugar levels in blood, similar to what we were taught before that carbohydrates were sugars as well as starch. The body reacts to fructose in a similar way like it handles alcohol, which is it is a toxin. When we inject anything with fructose, at minimum 90% is processed by the liver. By overriding the normal metabolic pathway by going straight to the liver. There, fructose will be transformed into pyruvate and then citrate. It is later converted into VLDL (low-density lipoprotein). VLDL is responsible for the accumulation of fat around the abdomen (beer belly and soda belly). Certain citrates are converted into Free Fatty Acids as well and could be absorbed into muscles of your body and lead to muscle insulin resistance. However, not all citrates are able to get out of the liver, that can lead to fat accumulation within the liver that are which is known as fatty liver diseases. It also makes Uric Acid when metabolized, which can cause high blood pressure, which can lead to hypertension.

Type 1 Diabetes Type 2 diabetes

It destroys beta cells within the pancreas. As a result, the pancreas is unable to produce insulin. Insulin resistance is the ineffective utilization of insulin in the body is known as insulin resistance.

Unrelated to excess body mass. It's associated with excess body weight

Autoimmune disease, low sensitivity to insulin. It isn't cutting down sugar levels like it is supposed to.

Every person who suffers from type 1 diabetes is required to inject insulin. Hence, those who are insulin dependent often require insulin injections to prevent hyperglycemia(excessive blood sugar)

Ketone levels higher at the time of initial diagnosis. Treatment is with medication and injections. Possible to reduce

If we refer to diabetes, we usually refer to type 2 diabetes that is related to type 1 as an uncommon condition.

There are various classifications for the most recommended type 2 diabetes are

Thiazolidinediones (Actos) targets the PPAR Gamma receptors, which are involved in the way the body stores fat as well as processes glucose. They could cause the body to store an excess amount of fluid. This may result in swelling (edema) as well as the weight to increase. This extra fluid may cause more problems or cause heart failing. Other side effects include bladder cancer, fractured bones, diabetic eye diseases that causes swelling at the behind of the eye (macular edema) liver issues as well as sore throats, muscle irritation, respiratory infections of the upper airways.

Sulfonylureas (Glimperide) These sulfonylureas attach to beta cells within the pancreas, thereby increasing the quantity of insulin that is produced. The most common side effects include weight increase (wherever there's insulin it is fat) and the condition known as hypoglycemia (low blood pressure)

Sodium-glucose Transporter (SGLT) two inhibitors (invokana) can affect kidney's capacity to absorb glucose back into blood, which results in a decrease in the blood sugar levels. The body flushes out excess glucose via urine. It can cause Hypoglycemia (low blood pressure) and Urinary tract infections (excess glucose passing through the urine) as well as liver damage too.

DPP-4 inhibitors (Januvia) block the natural enzyme in the body DDP-4. DDP-4 is a protein found throughout the body that plays a part in the immune system, and is involved in cell-to-cell interaction as well as apoptosis (bad cells dying). DDP-4 is also a blocker of the intestinal hormones known as incretins. which stimulate insulin, and decrease glycogen levels in the liver. It can cause pancreatitis (inflamed pancreas) as well as skin reactions, signs of flu, and intestinal issues.

Biguanides (metformin) are responsible for stopping the liver's capacity to produce glucose using amino acids and proteins. They do this and also stimulating the enzyme (AMPK) that helps cells respond better to insulin and process glucose within the blood. Biguanides such as metformin have been proven to trigger the condition known as lactic acidosis. The cause of lactic acidosis is the accumulation of lactate (L-lactate) in kidneys that drastically reduces the pH of your body. Biguanides trigger an increase in the production rate and a decrease in the elimination of lactate, resulting in elevated levels of cellular lactate. They can also cause the reduction in b12 levels and flatulence, as well as diarrhea, fatigue, sleepiness and joint pain.

The number of patients who were required to treat type 2 diabetes in the past five years of treatment using prescribed medications was: no one was helped (prevented stroke) None were assisted (prevented the death) None were assisted(stopped heart attacks) and none of them were helped (prevented heart attack), to prevent kidney failing) and one in 250 patients were assisted (prevented Amputation of a limb)

The reported amount of be harmed was 1 in 6 in 5 years (severe hypoglycemia hospitalization was required).

TCM Diabetes

The term "Xiao-ke" is used in Traditional Chinese Medicine Diabetes is called Xiao-ke "wasting and drinking". Diabetes can be classified into three components of the organ-meridian systems: middle, upper and lower. The higher form of diabetes is characterised by excessive thirst, while the middle type is associated with a high level of appetite, and the bottom is characterized by the frequent use of urinary frequency. It is interesting that these are also the primary signs for diagnosing diabetes coming from the western perspective. The Triple Warmer found in TCM is one of the Yang meridians of the fire organ. The Triple Warmer is accountable for production of "essential energy" that is composed of two kinds: the nourishment component includes "Ying Ch'i" (blood) that circulates through meridians. The other is the defense aspect "Wei Ch'i" (lymph fluid) which is absorbed by joints, muscles bone, skin, and the bones. It defends your body from attacks from external pressures. The general position of the Triple Warmer throughout the body lies in the stomach, throat and the pelvic area.

The upper burning strengthens the meridians of the heart and lung, and transfers the energy essential to Ying as well as Wei. Middle burning balances the stomach and the spleen. Therefore, it's accountable for the elimination of nutrients from food items and processing of food. Lower burning is responsible for harmonizing the kidneys, liver in the bladder and the intestine and plays a role in the intake of nutrients, removal of waste, the storage of energy, as well as reproductive roles. The triple warmer system forming one of the Yang part, Yin deficiency is often connected to Diabetes (Xiao-ke) within TCM. The signs of a Yin deficiency are weak, fatigue, and a dull complexion. Two other factors that contribute to the Xiao-ke diagnostic are a poor food habits (large portions of sugar, carbs and greasy foods, as well as fried, oily along with hot drinks and alcohol) as well as emotional stress (worry and anxiety, depression).

TCM herbal remedies for diabetes

Chinese CucumberChinese Cucumber Trichosanthes The root (Tian Hua Fen) has been utilized over the years to provide its cooling effect. The cause of diabetes is believed to be an imbalance of body heat which is why this helps balance the warmth. Chinese Cucumber tastes sweet and its primary ingredient is cold. It is absorbed into the stomach and lung meridians. Its primary function is to flush excess thirst and heat it also increases stomach and intestinal fluids. Its primary function is to treat the middle burn of diabetes. In nations like China as well as Taiwan trichosanthes is one of one of the most popular herbs for treating diabetes. Trichosanthes are known to be hypoglycemic in tests on animals as well as the capacity to boost the tolerance to glucose.

Poriaor Fu Ling (Poria cocos) is a medicinal mushroom that has been employed in TCM. One of the most frequently employed herbs used for Yin. It is it is a Yin herb, it helps in reducing the retention of fluids, Poria regulates metabolism, and also improves the kidneys and bladder. It also aids in the circulation of Ch'i in the Triple Warmer, which is important to the vital meridians. When studying animal models that were conducted with patients suffering from type 2 diabetes Poria was found to have a hypoglycemic impact. The main ingredient that are present in Poria is dehydrotrametenolic acid. It was found to influence its PPA R gamma receptor (which plays a role in the sensitivity to insulin) similar to a more natural form of Thiazolidinediones.

China Licorice RootChinese Licorice Root Kan Tsao (Glycyrrhizae Uralensis) is among the extensively utilized plant in China. The herb is helpful to all 12 meridians specifically for the Spleen Stomach as well as the Lungs. Chinese Licorice has been associated as balancing the middle burn portion of the three warmer meridians. Also known as the ultimate cleanser, Chinese licorice cleans the blood and body of excessive toxic substances. Due to its cleansing properties, Chinese licorice has been utilized to control blood sugar levels inside the body. One of the ingredients found in Chinese Licorice is called isoliquiritigenin that has been proven to stop the rise in fat levels and lifestyle-related obesity as well as fat liver disease, as well as type 2 diabetes by stopping the activation of NLRP3 which is a protein that has been linked with diabetes.

Ayurveda/ Rasayana Diabetes

The term used to describe diabetes in Ayurveda texts is Prameha which is a combination of 'pra', meaning abundance, and 'meha' translating to urine. Prameha is distinguished by a high level of kidney function (in volume and frequency) as well as Turbidity (the discoloration of fluids with a large number of sediments). The three doshas vata pitta and kapha are in the grip of Prameha. At the beginning, Kapha (which controls bile and fat, and can be affected by excessive sweets such as carbs) can be over-exerted, thereby leading to Kaphaja Prameha (pre-diabetes). The progression continues until a reduction in Kapha. Pitta is then predominant, and regulates blood flow, leading to Pittaja Prameha (acute diabetes). In the future, it is possible to lose of Pitta. The process ends with Vata is a vital organ that transports nutrients out of the body through urine. It can lead to Vataja Prameha (chronic diabetes).

Signs of Prameha

Kaphaja Pittaja Vataja

Stuffy nose Extreme thirst Excessive appetite

The feeling of laziness is a heavy chest

anorexia, anemia and insomnia

The excessive salivation causes pain in the bladder and penis regions shakes

nausea Burning sensations, burning sensations

constipation, cough and diarrhea

Insomnia resulting from excessive acid build-up Dyspnea (shortness of breath)

The study of Ayurveda there are three different kinds of Prameha (Diabetes):

1.) Prabhuta Mootrata- prameha is associated with frequent urination.

2.) Avila Mootrata- prameha is associated with the turbidity (cloudiness) from urine.

3.) Madhumeha- associated with the presence of glucose (sugar) in urine.

There are around 20 distinct routes that Prameha can be classified into within the body via the urine flow. Each of these pathways comes with been given a name, and it affects on the three doshas. Kapha has a variety of Pramehas. Pitta is home to 6 different pramehas and Vata is home to 4 types of pramehas.

Kapha (pre diabetes) Prameha:

Name of Prameha Name of Prameha is equivalent to the name that appears Urinary tract

Udakameha Hydruria Urine appears colorless as water, has a high flow, and feels cold

Ikshuvalikameha Glycosuria Urine is sugar-based that is cloudy and sweet and it resembles water made of sugar

Sandrameha Chyluria When lymphatic circulation is disturbed, it can cause chyle to leak into kidneys as well as the urine, which causes urine to appear as white as milk. Urine is extremely viscous.

Sandra Prasadmeha's Urine somewhat dilute with glucose and is semi-viscous

Shukrameha There is no similar name. Urine is chalky white, and body hairs get excited when the process of passing urine.

Shukrameha Spermaturia Urine is sperm-rich the urine looks as thick

The Sheetameha Phosturia Urine color is cold, white and it is sweet in be savour

Siktameha Graveluria Like particles of sand in the urine, a sign of kidney stones

Shanairmeha Oliguria Urine flow becomes slower and the output becomes difficult to achieve.

Lalameha Pyuria Urine has pus or white blood cells which is a indication of UTI and urine gum similar

Pitta (acute diabetes) Prameha:

Name of Prameha Name of Prameha is equivalent to the name that appears Urinary tract

Kalameha Melanuria Urine contains melanin Urine color ranges between black and orange the color

Nilameha Indigouria Urine appears to be blue in color

Raktameha Hematuria Blood found in the urine. Urine appears to be red.

Manjishthameha Hemoglobinuria Urine looks as pink, and the urine smells foul.

Haridrameha Urobilinuria Urine is yellow-colored, with a strong scent can cause burning sensations.

Ksharmeha Alkaluria Urine which is somewhat acidic has become alkaline

Vata (Chronic Diabetes) Prameha:

Name of Prameha Name of Prameha is equivalent to the name that appears Urinary tract

Vasameha Lipuria Urine has a yellowish hue Urine is a source of the lipids (fats/vasa)

Majjameha Myelouria Urine is made up of bone Marrow (majja) The urine appears similar to nerve tissue.

The volume of urine in Hastimeha Diabetes Insipidus is huge, and it contains lymph (lasika)

Madhumeha Madhumeha Mellitus (type 2.) Urine is cloudy, sweet and light in color. The essence that the human organ (Oja) is losing

The best instance of the relationship between Ayurveda and body could be Pitta Prameha Haridrameha (Urobilinuria). The body's the urobolin (a chemical which makes urine yellow) is produced by the intestines. Urobolin comes as a result produced by Bilirubin that is created in the liver as it degrades the old blood vessels. Bilrubin is found in the bile and it is brownish/yellowish colored. Urobilinuria results from the inability of liver cells to eliminate away from circulation the urobilin pumped into the liver through the blood. Urobolin gets into kidneys' circulation and then is eliminated in urine. If the accumulation of urobilin is excessive in the intestines, harm to the liver could happen. This is a clear indication that this could be an example of Pitta imbalance. Pitta regulates blood flow as well as its roles in Ayurveda the philosophy. If your liver and blood isn't functioning properly, the first indicator is a yellowish urine released.

Ayurveda/Rasayana herbs for Diabetes

Fenugreek (Trigonella foenum-graecum) isn't a plant however it is a legume which is used in Ayurveda medical practice and also for cooking in India for many years. The seeds of fenugreek are even discovered among the remains of graves of Egyptians in the ancient pyramids. Fenugreek can slow down the absorption rate of glucose and other simple carbohydrates because of its fiber-rich content. An investigation into the effects of fenugreek seeds in patients suffering from type 2 diabetes produced positive outcomes. The seeds of fenugreek were immersed into hot water, and then given over a period of 8 weeks. The FBS levels (fasting blood sugar) as well as the TG level (triglycerides) and the VLDL-C levels (very low density cholesterol in lipoproteins) have been reduced (25 percent, 30 percent and 365% and 365% respectively) (Kassaian N in 2009). Fenugreek seeds are rich in calcium, iron, potassium and copper. They also contain selenium, manganese, zinc and niacin. They also contain all B vitamins minus B12, as well as Vitamins A as well as C. It also contains polysaccharides, such as saponins tannins, hemicellulose, and pectin. They have been proven to decrease LDL through preventing cholesterol from absorption in the colon. Fenugreek is a rich source of the amino acid 4 hydroxyisoleucene that reduces the intake of glucose within the intestinal tract, thereby lowering blood sugar levels of diabetics.

Indian Plum/Jamun (Syzygium jambolensis) Jamun is a fruit that grows in the summer and can be that is found throughout India as well as Asia. Jamun has been utilized to for treating diabetes in Ayurveda for a long time. Jamun is rich in carotene, iron, folic acid calcium and magnesium. It also contains potassium and phosphorus as well as phytonutrients and antioxidants as well as Vitamin C. These seeds have glucoside jamboline, and ellagic acid that inhibits the process of converting starch to sugar and thus regulating the blood sugar level (J. Giri, 1985). Additionally, it has four times as much Vitamin C as an orange. Vitamin C is an effective antioxidant that helps to reduce LDL in the body, that is involved in the development of diabetes.

Bitter Gourd (Karela)Bitter Gourd (Karela) Melon (Momordica Charantia) makes up the Cucurbitaceae family, and is native to Asia,

South America, India and East Africa. Bitter Gourd is a great remedy for violating Kapha as well as Pitta doshas. The flavor is sour and bitter, which is its name. A cup of bittermelon contains more than 140% of the suggested daily dose of Vitamin C. Bitter Melon also has magnesium, zinc, potassium manganese, iron folate, copper, calcium and all B vitamins, with the exception of B12, as well as Vitamin A. The most potent phytonutrient that are found within bitter melon are a polypeptide found to reduce the levels of glucose in both animals and human beings when consumed (Tayyab F 2012). The plant "insulin" is a molecule that mimics the actions of insulin within the body, which reduces blood sugar levels within the body. Bitter melon is also a source of Charantin, a chemical which is found only within the plant kingdom. Charantin boosts the absorption of glucose and glycogen production within the cells of the muscles, liver as well as fatty tissues. In an 8-week research in mice with type 2 diabetes given bitter melon results revealed a dramatic reduction in the non-fasting blood glucose levels, insulin resistance, and plasma glucose intolerance. insulin resistance. (Hsien-Yi Wang, 2014)

The use of Alkaline or Electric herbs to treat Diabetes

HuerequeHuereque Coyote Melon (Ibervillea sonorae) is utilized throughout South America to treat Diabetes. Coyote melon is a member of the Cucurbitaceae or Gourd family of vegetable and is closely related to cucumber. It is a source of valuable phytonutrients and tannins. One of the phytonutrients that are plentiful in the melon of the coyote is Gallic Acid. Gallic acid is a chemical that is found in plant tissues and functions as an antioxidant in nature. Gallic acid has been proven by tests that it has positive effects on glucose levels as well as insulin sensitivity. It does this by decreasing the levels of fasting and normal glucose as well as increasing the sensitivity of insulin (Khanh V., 2015).The Roots of Coyote Melon also contain dichloromethane (DCM) that has been observed to reduce fasting blood sugar levels and increase the levels of insulin in serum and improve oral glucose tolerance (Zhaoxia Liu, 2013).

The Nopal Cactus/Prickly Pear (Opuntia) is a type of cactus that is native of North as well as South America. Nopal is among the minerals-rich food sources that exist on earth. Nopal is rich in calcium, copper and iron as well as manganese, magnesium, phosphorous as well as potassium, selenium zinc, sodium, and all B vitamins with the exception of B12 Vitamin A C and E. The other components include pectin, fiber, and 17 amino acids out of eight of which is essential amino acid. Nopal is used to combat diabetes for a lengthy time throughout Central America and by the American Indians. Nopal is known to dramatically reduce blood glucose levels in diabetics with type 2 diabetes (Gutierrez

1998). A different study gave people suffering from Type 2 diabetes with a high carb breakfast, with or with and without Nopal as an ingredient. Results showed that Nopal can reduce serum glucose, insulin levels, as well as plasma glucose-dependent insulinotropic Peptide (GIP) peak levels in addition to increasing antioxidant activity among people suffering from Type 2 diabetes (J 2014).

Nettle or Stinging Nettle (Urtica Dioica) is a slender herbaceous perennial that is a wild green across the globe. Nettle is among the plants with the highest concentration of nutrients found in nature. Nettle contains four times the quantity of Vitamin C against one moderately sized orange. Nettle also has Vitamins A B1, B1, K calcium, potassium ferric oxide (non-hemoglobin iron). In addition, agglutinin alkaloids, acetylcholine and as well as butyric acid Terminalia caffeic acid carbonic acid, choline histamine, coumaric acids, theophyllin, formic acids, coproporphyrin, lectin and ermin. the linolenic and linoleic acids as well as palmitic acid, xanthophyll quercetin, quinic acid serotonin, stigmasterol Terpenes, violaxanthin and succinic acids in the chemical composition (1. Ayan AK, 2006). 30% - 40 percent Nettle is mostly protein, and is also rich in fiber. Fiber aids in controlling blood pressure and digestion. The study found that nettle improved the sensitivity of insulin and stimulated glucose metabolism in muscles of the skeletal. These results suggest that nettle can be a useful supplement to metabolic diseases including the condition of insulin resistance (Diana N. Obanda, 2016,).

Other herbal remedies for diabetes

Afara/Limba/Ofram/Korina (Terminalia superba) - is a tree that is native to the West Africa area and has been used as a medicinal remedy for centuries. The tree's bark is usually chewed, or made into tea. The bark is rich in gallic acid as well as the methyl gallate that have demonstrated significant capacity to reduce the level of glucose. Additionally, extracts of alcohol from the bark have also been proven to have anti-diabetic and vasorelaxant actions. A study on rats with diabetes showed extracts of the Limba tree are able to help reverse hyperglycemia, thereby having anti-diabetic qualities (Kamtchouing P. 2006).

Neem (Azadirachta indica) - is a tree of green that belongs to South Asia countries. According to Indian mythology it is believed that the tree is divine and made from nectar drops emanating from the heavens. Neem originates from Sanskrit Nimba, which means to grant health (Puri 1999). Neem oil has been proven to have its ability to reduce sugar levels and is extensively used in India to treat diabetes. The cause of diabetes is the pancreas becoming weak and may lead to pancreatic cancer. The oil of Neem contains nimbolide. during a laboratory study, nimbolide decreased the ability of pancreatic cancerous cells to increase their growth and metabolism by 70%. Thus, cancer cells were unable to grow. Cancerous cells were to be attacked from every angle the use of an ingredient called nimbolide (Subramani R, 2016,).

Aloe Vera (Aloe barbadensis miller) is the first recorded humans using aloe vera is discovered in the Ebers Papyrus (an Egyptian medical scroll) from the 16th (Amar Surjushe in 2008). The origins of the plant are in Africa which dates back to 600 years ago, but it can currently be seen throughout the world. The aloe plant is rich in Vitamins A C, E B12, folic acids, copper, calcium, chromium selenium, magnesium, manganese, potassium and zinc, sodium and sugars (glucose and fructose) as well as hormones. It also contains 20 of 22 amino acids as well as seven of the eight essential amino acids, as well as various phytonutrients. The aloe vera plant has demonstrated a an impressive reduction in blood glucose levels. It has is also proven to decrease HbA1c (Minh Q Ngo D and Sachin A Shah, 2010,).

Rosemary (Rosmarinus officinalis) as well as Greek Oregano (Origanum Vulgare) as well as Mexican Oregano (Lippia Graveolens) These are the herbs that the majority of users are familiar with, yet very few are aware of their therapeutic properties. The plants contain phytonutrients that are beneficial as well as flavonoids. Gallic acid was discovered in both of these plants in high levels. Gallic acid is known to have glucose-lowering impacts on our bodies and has been shown to block enzymes that are involved in the secretion of insulin and signals (Allyson M Bower (2014)).

Chapter 7: Common Modern Ailments and Their Chinese Herbal Treatments

Chinese herb medicine has been in use for a number of years for treating a diverse range of illnesses as well as its efficacy is well documented throughout the history of medicine. Nowadays, a variety of modern illnesses are treated by Chinese herbalism and this ancient treatment technique is now being increasingly acknowledged as an effective instrument for treating the most common health issues of modern times.

The most frequent illnesses that Chinese herbs can successfully combat is anxiety and stress. Stress is an integral aspect of our lives, but when it gets persistent, it could cause damage to the physical and mental wellbeing of our patients. Chinese herb medicine provides many ingredients and formulas that aid in reducing anxiety and stress by creating an atmosphere of peace and peace. The most frequently utilized herbs include ashwagandha which is well-known for its capacity to relieve stress and increase peace, as well as passionflower, that is utilized to relax your mind and induce sleep.

A different modern condition which can be addressed using Chinese herbs is exhaustion and fatigue. There are many people who suffer with fatigue and exhaustion that is chronic which is often the result of the combination of causes like stress, inadequate diet and inadequate exercising. Chinese herbs are many tonic plants that help improve energy levels and increase vitality like ginseng, for example. It is believed to be a potent tonic herb which can boost endurance and energy astragalus can help to improve the immune system and boost general well-being.

Chinese herbs can aid in the treatment of problems with digestion, such as constipation, bloating, and diarrhea. The majority of digestive problems can be due to a variety of elements like unhealthy diet, stress as well as a absence of exercise. Chinese herbal medicine provides many ingredients and formulas that assist in the regulation of the digestive tract and help promote healthful digestion. A few of the most widely employed herbs are ginger, well-known for its capacity to calm stomachs and aid in healthy digestion and licorice which is employed to ease the digestion tract and decrease inflammation.

A common modern-day ailment that is treatable using Chinese herb medicine are migraines and headaches. Migraines and headaches could be result of a range of reasons, such as tension, diet and stress as well as a lack of sleep. Chinese herbal medicine provides various herbal remedies and formulations that aid in relieving headaches and migraines by decreasing inflammation as well as boosting circulation of blood to the head. The most frequently utilized herbs are fever few that is utilized to lower inflammation and increase healthy blood flow to the brain as well as white willow bark that is renowned as a pain reliever.

Chinese herbs can aid in the treatment of breathing problems like asthma, bronchitis, or allergies. These respiratory issues are usually due to a mix of causes, including unhealthy diet, stress as well as exposure to environmental toxins. Chinese herbal medicine provides numerous herbal remedies and formulations that aid in relieving respiratory issues through reducing inflammation as well as promoting the health of your lungs. The most frequently employed herbs are Phaedra that is renowned as a potent herb that can open the lungs, and boost the function of breathing, as well as mahuang, which helps for reducing inflammation and promoting the health of your lungs.

While reading this chapter, picture that you are picking herbs out of the fields, as well as the process of preparing the herbs to drink.

Feel the warmth of herbal teas or compresses that eases your pain and that sense of wellbeing and balance which it brings. Chinese herbalism is an effective and natural method to combat common modern illnesses as well as an excellent tool for those who wants to boost your health and wellbeing.

It is important to remember that although Chinese herbs may be beneficial in the treatment of numerous modern illnesses however, it's important to seek out a licensed practitioner prior to using any herb or other formulas. The practitioner is capable of creating a customized treatment program based on your particular requirements and your health history and is able to keep track of the progress of your treatment and adjust when needed.

In addition, Chinese herbal medicine can be utilized in conjunction with other treatments including Western medical treatment or Acupuncture. The practitioner will be capable of advising you on the appropriate treatment that is appropriate for you considering any other treatment or medication you are receiving.

In the end, Chinese herbal medicine offers an efficient and safe method to address a wide range of common diseases. From anxiety and stress, to headaches, fatigue and respiratory issues, Chinese herbal medicine offers many different herbs and formulas to assist in improving your the health of your body and improve overall well-being. When you work with a certified doctor, you'll be able to develop an individual treatment plan which will ease your symptoms, and help promote peace and harmony within the body, mind as well as your spirit.

The Principles of Chinese Herbal Therapy

Chinese herb therapy is a fundamental component of the traditional Chinese medical practice, and is founded upon a set of fundamentals that have been refined through many years of experience. The principles underlying these are the idea that the mind, body as well as the soul are inextricably linked and that healing truly requires taking care of each one of them.

One of the main tenets that underlie Chinese herbal treatment is the notion of the concept of balance. In traditional Chinese medical practices, the human body is constantly in perpetual change. Health is dependent upon the equilibrium of vital energy in the body called Qi. If Qi flows freely and is balanced and in balance, the body is in the best well-being. If Qi is restricted or is out of alignment the body can suffer and illness may be a result. Chinese herb therapy aims to restore harmony within the body, by correcting the imbalances underlying that are responsible for the condition.

A further principle that is central to Chinese herb therapy lies in the notion of synergy.

Chinese herbal therapy is founded on the application of formulas for herbal use, which comprise a variety of herbal remedies that are tailored specifically to the requirements of each patient. The formulas are created to target the specific characteristics of each person and help promote balance and harmony within the body. Utilizing multiple herbs in formulas allows that the various herbs be used together to create an impact synergistic to be more that the total of its components.

Individualization is also a major factor for Chinese traditional medicine. Every patient is different, and each illness is distinct. Chinese herbs recognize this fact by customizing formulations for herbal medicine to the particular needs of each particular patient. The approach is based on not just the individual's symptoms but also their entire health history, constitution and their lifestyle. This ensures that treatments are tailored to each individual patient's needs, and it is more efficient.

Another characteristic in Chinese herb therapy involves that it relies on natural ingredients. Chinese herbal therapy relies on the usage of natural substances made from minerals, plants and even animals. They are thought to work in harmony with our bodies and have less risk of causing negative side effects than synthetic substances. They are typically employed in their natural forms like the root or stem, leaves or even flowers. They are processed in a variety of methods, like fermenting or drying, in order to improve their medicinal qualities.

The idea of gradualness also plays a role for Chinese herb therapy. Chinese herb therapy is aware the healing process is being a gradual process, and it is crucial to make smaller steps to heal. Formulas and herbs are utilized in small amounts, and gradual increase as the health improves. This helps avoid the occurrence of adverse reactions as well as allowing the body to slowly adjust to the treatments.

Chapter 8: Herbs for Immune Support and Inflammation

Chinese herb medicine has many different herbs that are used to aid in the development of immunity and lessen inflammation. They have been utilized over the years to help prevent and treat ailments and are well-known as a way to increase the body's defenses naturally and help to heal.

One of the most widely employed herbs used to boost immunity is Astragalus. It is a herb that has been praised as a powerful herb that can boost the immune system as well as improve general well-being. It's regarded as a tonic herb. This means it works in replenishing and strengthening the vital energy of your body also known as Qi. Astragalus is commonly utilized in formulations to combat colds and flu as well as for promoting healing following an disease. In the form of a tea or a decoction it assists in boosting digestion and decrease fatigue.

A different herb commonly utilized to support the immune system is Echinacea. The herb is known for its capacity to boost the immune system, and decrease inflammation. The herb is commonly used for treating and preventing respiratory illnesses such as the flu and colds. Echinacea is also renowned for its capacity to ease inflammation as well as promote healing of the body. If consumed in the form of tea or in a tincture, it's frequently used to treat coughing, sore throat as well as other signs of influenza and colds.

Reishi mushroom is a different powerful herb commonly utilized in order to boost immunity and decrease inflammation. It is renowned as a powerful booster of your immune system's strength, lower inflammation and boost general well-being. The herb is commonly used to treat and prevent many different diseases, such as the autoimmune diseases, cancer as well as viral diseases. Reishi mushroom is consumed in capsules, tinctures and even in tea form, and is renowned for its distinct earthy taste.

Ginger is a different herb that is used extensively to help reduce inflammation and strengthen our immune system. It is renowned for its capacity to relax stomach pain and encourage healthy digestion. Also, it is known for its anti-inflammatory properties. In fact, it can be used to help reduce inflammation of muscles and joints. It is also utilized to treat and prevent the flu and cold. Ginger can be consumed as tea, mixed into meals or used in a dietary supplement.

Turmeric is a second herb commonly utilized in order to lessen inflammation and boost your immune system. The herb is well-known for its anti-inflammatory properties, and is frequently utilized to help reduce swelling in muscles and joints. Turmeric is also renowned for its capacity to improve the immune system as well as improve general well-being. It is typically utilized as a spice for the kitchen or used as a supplement as a supplement. Its bright yellow hue is a visible illustration of its powerful anti-inflammatory capabilities.

Herbs for Stress and Anxiety Management

Anxiety and stress are both common concerns that impact a large number of people in the present, and Chinese herbs offer many different herbs that are used to alleviate and manage these issues. They have been utilized throughout history to help relax as well as calm your mind and boost overall health.

The most widely employed herbs in managing anxiety and stress is Ashwagandha. The herb is widely known as a remedy to decrease anxiety and stress as well as promote relaxation. It's regarded as an adaptogenic plant, which means it assists the body in adapting to stresses and improves the equilibrium. Ashwagandha is commonly utilized in formulations that help lower anxiety levels and boost general well-being. If consumed in tea form or supplement to a diet, it helps increase sleep and decrease fatigue.

Passionflower is yet another plant which is widely used in the management of anxiety and stress. It is renowned for its capacity to soothe your mind and induce a peaceful sleep. It's often utilized for relieving the symptoms of insomnia and anxiety it can be ingested in tea form or the form of a tincture. The stems and leaves the plant are unique and complex shape that could be used as an image of the ability of this herb to calm and relax the mind.

The Skullcap herb is employed to decrease anxiety and stress in addition to enhancing sleep. It is well-known as a herb that can calm the mind and induce relaxation. The herb is frequently used to alleviate symptoms of insomnia, anxiety as well as restlessness. The Skullcap herb can be consumed by drinking tea or using it as a tincture. its delicate blue flowers could provide an illustration of the herb's relaxing properties.

Lemon Balm is another herb that is frequently used to aid in the management of anxiety and stress. It is renowned for its capacity to encourage peace and enhance overall wellbeing. It's often utilized for relieving symptoms of insomnia, anxiety and even insomnia. It can be ingested by drinking tea or in an tincture. Its aroma is fresh and refreshing. It can be used as a visual reminder of its ability to boost mood and decrease stress.

Jujube is often employed for stress and anxiety managing. The herb is renowned as a potent stimulant to increase peace and enhance overall wellbeing. It's often utilized to alleviate the symptoms of insomnia, anxiety and anxiousness. Jujube is a drinkable tea that can be taken in tea form or as a tincture. Jujube's sweetness and nourishment could serve as a visualization of the herb's capacity to soothe the mind and create peace and wellbeing.

Valerian is often utilized for stress and anxiety control. The herb is well-known for its capacity to induce relaxation and enhance sleep. It's often utilized in order to ease symptoms of insomnia, anxiety and agitation. Valerian is a drinkable herb that can be taken in tea form or as an tincture. Its particular root structure is able to provide a visual illustration of the herb's capacity to relax and soothe the mind.

Chapter 9: Herbs for Digestive Health

Chinese herbal medicine provides many different herbs which can be utilized in order to improve digestion overall health. They have been utilized over the centuries to enhance digestion, ease stomach pain and boost overall wellbeing.

One of the most frequently utilized herbs to aid in digestion is Ginger. It is renowned for its ability to relax stomach pain and improve digestion. Additionally, it has its anti-inflammatory properties. In fact, it is frequently utilized to help reduce discomfort in the gastrointestinal tract. It is widely used for relieving symptoms like nausea, constipation or stomach discomfort. Ginger can be drunk in the form of tea, as a cooking ingredient and eaten in a supplement. If you drink it, the warming and sour aroma could bring sensations of comfort and relaxation, imagining its ability to calm stomach.

Another plant that is widely employed to treat digestive issues is Licorice. Licorice is renowned as a soothing herb that can soothe the digestive tract as well as reduce inflammation. This herb is frequently utilized to treat symptoms associated with indigestion, stomach ulcers and various digestive problems. Licorice may be ingested by drinking tea or using it as a supplement. its sweet and soothing flavor may bring about feelings of balance and wellbeing.

Peppermint is often utilized to boost digestion. It is well-known as a soothing herb that can soothe stomachs, ease inflammation and ease the symptoms of stomach and indigestion discomfort. Peppermint is a drinkable herb that can be used in tea form or as the form of a tincture. The fresh and uplifting scent may induce feelings of balance and wellbeing.

Turmeric is yet another plant widely utilized for digestion well-being. The herb is known for its anti-inflammatory properties, and frequently used to decrease intestinal inflammation. Turmeric is also renowned for its capacity to boost overall well-being and health. The most common way to consume it is to spice up cooking or in supplements, as well as its vibrant yellow hue could be an image of its anti-inflammatory qualities.

Fennel is often utilized to treat digestive issues. The herb is well-known for its capacity to relax the stomach, alleviate gas and bloating, and enhance digestion in general. Fennel is a drinkable herb that can be taken in the form of tea or an tincture. Its distinctive and delicate form is a good visual representation of its capacity to boost digestion.

Herbs for Cardiovascular Health

Chinese herb medicine has an array of herbal remedies which can be utilized in order to boost and enhance heart health. They have been utilized since the beginning of time to increase circulation, reduce blood pressure, and boost general well-being.

One of the most frequently employed herbs in the field of heart wellbeing is Hawthorn. It is renowned for its capacity to boost circulation as well as lower blood pressure. It's regarded as tonic, which means it aids in replenishing and strengthen your vital energy of the body, referred to as Qi. Hawthorn is frequently utilized in formulations that help fight heart disease and to improve the overall health of your heart. In the form of tea, it can help in boosting digestion and reducing fatigue. The bright red berries and the thorny leaves can be used as visual reminders of the plant's capacity to boost and safeguard the heart.

Another plant that is widely utilized to improve the health of your heart is Garlic. It is well-known as a great way to decrease cholesterol levels as well as improve circulation. Also, it is known for its anti-inflammatory properties. Garlic can be used in reducing inflammation of the heart and lungs. Garlic can be taken as a food supplement or added to food preparation as well as its sour aroma could be an illustration of its capability to boost the health of your cardiovascular system.

Cayenne peppers are also widely employed to enhance heart health. The herb is renowned for its capacity to boost blood flow, decrease blood pressure and ease symptoms associated with angina. Cayenne pepper is consumed as a cooking spice or used as a supplement and its bright red hue could be visual evidence of its capacity to boost the health of your cardiovascular system.

Chapter 10: Herbs for Women's Health

Chinese herbal medicine provides many different herbs that are used to aid and enhance women's overall health. The use of these herbs has been practiced since the beginning of time to regulate menstrual cycle and relieve the pain of menstrual cramps, and boost overall health.

The most widely utilized herbs to treat women's health is Dong Qi. The herb is well-known as a remedy to control menstrual cycles and ease the pain of menstruation. It's considered to be a tonic plant, which means it can help replenish and boost your body's vital energy known as Qi. Dong Quai is commonly employed in formulas to control menstrual flow and enhance overall fertility health. If consumed in the form of tea, it can help in boosting digestion and reducing fatigue. The delicate roots and stem may serve as a symbolic symbol of the herb's power to provide nourishment and support to the reproductive system of females.

A different herb commonly utilized for the health of women includes Black Cohosh. The herb is renowned as a remedy for painful menstrual cramps and control the menstrual cycle. Also, it is well-known for its capacity to reduce symptoms associated with menopausal change including hot flashes and mood fluctuations. Black Cohosh can be consumed in tea form or used as a supplement. its deep, dark-colored roots is an image of its capability to regulate menstrual cycles and boost overall health.

Red Raspberry Leaf is also often used to boost women's overall health. It is well-known as a remedy to control the menstrual cycle, ease the pain of menstrual cramps, and strengthen and prepare the uterus in preparation for the upcoming pregnancy. It is also known for its ability to tone and prepare the uterus for pregnancy. Raspberry Leaf is a drinkable in tea form, and the deep green leaves are an image of the herb's capability to nourishe and strengthen the female reproductive system.

Angelica can also be utilized to treat women's health. The herb is well-known for its capacity to regulate menstrual cycles, relieve menstrual cramps and cramps and enhance overall health of the reproductive system. The herb is also renowned as a remedy for menopausal symptoms like mood swings and hot flashes. Angelica is a drinkable herb that can be taken by drinking tea or using it as an addition to a diet, and its sturdy and tall stems as well as delicate white flowers could serve as visual evidence of its ability to help strengthen and protect the female reproductive system.

Motherwort is another herbal remedy which is widely used to improve women's wellbeing. It is renowned for its capacity to regulate the menstrual cycle, ease cramps and pain during menstruation as well as improve general health of the reproductive system. Also, it is known as a remedy for symptoms of menopausal, such as hot flashes, mood swings and so on. Motherwort is a drinkable herb that can be taken as in tea form or as concoction, and its tiny flowers are able to serve as a visual representation for its ability to help support and improve the reproductive system.

Herbs for Men's Health

Chinese herbal medicine has an array of herbal remedies which can be utilized in order to improve and support health for men. The use of these herbs has been practiced throughout history to enhance sexual performance, boost prostate health, and improve general well-being.

A popular and widely employed herbs for the health of men are Saw Palmetto. The herb is well-known as a potent herb that can improve sexual performance and improve prostate health. The herb is commonly utilized to treat the symptoms associated with an overly large prostate as well as improve urinary functions. Saw Palmetto can be consumed in a way as a supplement and its tiny, dark-colored fruits can function as an illustration of the ability of this herb to aid and enhance the male reproductive system.

A different herb commonly employed to treat men's health is the Horny Goat Weed. The herb is recognized as a potent ingredient that can improve sexual health and improve overall health. The herb is commonly used to treat the symptoms of erectile disorder and enhance overall sexual health. Horny goat weed may be taken as a supplement as well as its distinctive and complex leaves could be used as an image of the herb's capability to enhance sexual performance.

It is also utilized to boost men's health. The herb is renowned as a potent herb that can improve sexual functioning and improve overall health. The herb is frequently used to treat the symptoms of low libido as well as increase overall sexual well-being. It can be taken as a supplement and the small, sharp leaves are an image of the herb's capacity to enhance sexual performance.

Ginseng is often used in the treatment of male health. The herb is well-known as a potent herb that can improve sexual performance, improve overall health, and improve the level of energy. The herb is commonly employed to alleviate the symptoms of erectile disfunction, anxiety, fatigue and depression. Ginseng is a drinkable herb that can be taken as an herbal tea or as a supplement. its unique root structure may be used as a symbol of the plant's capacity to nourish and bolster the male body.

Epimedium is a second herb commonly utilized for health and wellness of males. It is renowned for its capacity to enhance sexual performance, improve general health, and improve performance levels.

The herb is frequently used to treat symptoms of erectile disorder and increase overall health of sexuality. Epimedium is a drink that can be taken in the form of a supplement. the delicate flower can act as a visual representation for its ability to enhance sexual health.

Chapter 11: Incorporating Chinese Herbs in Your Health Plan

Chinese herb medicine is an effective and natural method to enhance and sustain general health and wellbeing. The incorporation of Chinese herbal remedies into your daily regimen could provide an holistic method of healing that addresses not only issues but also health issues that are affecting the body.

Incorporating Chinese herbal remedies into your daily program, it's essential to consult with a certified professional who can develop an individual treatment program specific specifically to your requirements and health issues. An experienced doctor will consider your health history, symptoms as well as your overall health in order to identify the most effective herbal remedies to utilize and the right dosage.

If you are taking Chinese herbal remedies, it's essential to know that they may produce a cumulative effect, and can take time to get results. You must be perseverant and persistent in using the herbal supplements as directed by your doctor.

The most popular methods of consuming Chinese herbs is by making decoctions, which are an approach to boil the herbs in water in order to get their healing properties. This process allows for more concentrated concentration of the active components and is an effective method to consume the herb.

Another method of consuming Chinese herbs is by taking the tincture method, which is a liquid extract from the herb.

Tinctures are simple to consume and may be a better option to those with difficulty taking pills.

Chinese herbs may also be taken by taking capsules, pills, or granules. They are packaged in a convenient way, and easy to use, and may provide a great choice for those constantly on the move. These kinds of herbal remedies are typically used by those who struggle to remember to drink the herbal tea regularly.

It's also crucial to keep in mind that Chinese herbs are best used together with a balanced diet and a lifestyle. Consuming a balanced and healthy diet with plenty of vegetables, fruits along with whole grains, proteins that are lean can aid in the healing process and increase the efficacy of herb. Regular exercise, stress reduction strategies, and proper sleep are crucial for general health and wellbeing.

Safety and Precautions for Chinese Herbal Medicine

Chinese herb medicine is an safe and efficient type of medicine if used in a proper manner and under the supervision of a trained doctor. It is crucial to be aware that just like every type of medication, Chinese herbal remedies can cause negative effects, as well as interactions with other drugs.

Incorporating Chinese herbal remedies into your daily program, you need that you work with a licensed professional who has been trained on the proper use and security of Chinese herbal remedies. They'll consider any medical issues or allergies, as well as medications. that you might need to check that the prescribed herbs are safe to take.

Also, it is important to be aware that there are some exceptions to the rule that Chinese herbalism are safe for all. Certain herbs are not recommended for specific people, like mothers who are pregnant, which is why they should not be used. It is crucial to know that certain herbs can interact with other medication you're using, and it's essential to inform your doctor of any medicines you're currently using.

A further aspect to consider when it comes to safety is making sure that the plants you're using are high-quality and not contaminated. It is essential to buy herbal products from reliable sources, like licensed practitioners or dispensaries to make sure that the plants that you take have been proven to be safe and of high quality.

While reading this chapter, you can imagine yourself inside a lab, with a variety of plants and tools, imagining how herbs are tested carefully and scrutinized to confirm their safety and quality. Imagine how a trained doctor carefully assesses the condition of your body and medication prior to giving you a prescription, so that they can ensure that you're safe and the herbal remedies fit for you.

As a summary, Chinese herbal medicine is an safe and reliable method of treatment when utilized in a proper manner and under the supervision by a licensed practitioner. Working with a licensed practitioner, buying herbs from trusted sources and being aware of possible interaction and side effects You can be sure of the safe and efficient usage of Chinese herbal remedies in your daily treatment regimen.

The Future of Chinese Herbal Medicine

Chinese herbalism has been in use for centuries for improving health and well-being Its popularity is growing with increasing numbers of individuals seek out organic and natural forms of medical treatment. It is expected that the future for Chinese herbal medicine is promising as researchers continue to discover the benefits to health that can be gained from herbal remedies and their effectiveness to treat a myriad of illnesses.

A major and thrilling innovations in the field of Chinese herbology is the growing amount of scientific research uncovering the mechanisms of action as well as the potential advantages to health of these herbs. The research is conducted in order to discover how the herbs function on the molecular level as well as discover the active ingredients that are responsible for their therapeutic effects. The research helps prove the efficacy of Chinese herbal remedies in treating various diseases and also helps to integrate the traditional Chinese medical practices into mainstream health care.

A further significant development within the realm of Chinese herbology is the increased accessibility of high-quality standard herbal remedies. This is crucial because it guarantees that the herbal products are safe as well as effective and constant in their performance. This makes it much easier for physicians to prescribe appropriate herbs and users to choose the appropriate dose.

With the advancement of technology and advance, technology will continue to advance, and the next phase of Chinese herbal medicine is likely to be a more extensive usage of technology for supporting the practitioners as well as patients. Online consultations, telemedicine, as well as online databases of Chinese herbs are becoming increasingly widespread and provide more accessibility to Chinese herbs for patients.

Future prospects for Chinese herbal medicine is also characterized by growing interest in combining traditional Chinese treatment together with Western medical practices. The method, referred to as integrative therapy, may aid in bridging the gap between the different types of medical treatment and provide an integrated method of healthcare.

When you are reading this chapter, picture yourself inside a futuristic laboratory with the latest technology as well as cutting-edge equipment for research, envisioning the ways that researchers and practitioners come together to realize the potential of Chinese herbs. Imagine how technology will make the access to Chinese herbs more accessible and more efficient. Imagine how traditional Chinese medicine along with Western medical practices combine to provide an integrated approach to medical care.

The future of Chinese herbal medicine is looking positive as researchers continue to determine the possible advantages of these plants as the supply of top-quality, well-tested herb products grows. Technology integration as well as the integration of traditional Chinese medical practices along with Western medical practices will play a a important role in determining the direction of Chinese herb treatment.

Chapter 12: Chinese Medicine and Its History the Concept of Traditional Chinese Medicine

The genesis of Traditional Chinese Medicine (TCM) can be traced back to around 2300 years ago. It's a meticulously designed technique that focuses on healing yourself by using the traditional method. TCM relies on yin and Yang principles and is believed to be two separate forces that complement each other.

Yang is the dark feminine component. Yang is the masculine, light component. They are the basis of all universal manifestations. The yin-yang concept has roots in Chinese cultural traditions. Many significant Chinese concepts are ethically developed in tandem with the concept of yin-yang. It represents balance within the world.

The foundation of which Traditional Chinese Medicine derives the basis of its practice is Qi. Qi is the vital energy that circulates through every one of us. This energy-filled network binds every part of us. TCM employs a method which seeks to restore the flow of energy in the body.

Certain external and internal forces can let in negative qi within the body. The negative qi could cause harm to your body and can cause problems. TCM is the therapy that transforms harmful energy into healthy ones. Traditional Chinese Medicine works strictly in accordance with the natural law known as Tao. The Tao law says that humans are the same as his mind and cannot be separated even at the cost of.

TCM is determined to reach the status of "health for everyone." "Health to everyone" is a goal to provide equally good health care to all who need it, regardless of their personal circumstances. It is essential to make a pledge to provide an equal opportunity for all in health care. The health agendas must be adhered to with a great deal of dedication. This also means that the people have a good understanding of healthcare issues and understand that we have the ability to heal ourselves.

Yin-Yang

Let's discuss the concept of yin and Yang in more detail. Most of you know the symbol of black and white of the yin-yang concept. It is among the most popular philosophical theories in China.

We have discussed that it is the feminine aspect of both. It's closely associated with the Earth which is the dark silence and absorbence. Yang's masculine aspect creates heavenly, bright permeating, movable, and luminous elements. When it comes to the idea that is part of Traditional Chinese Medicine, yin and yang are the two elements that affect diverse organs. Let's discuss the elements that affect what organ.

Yin is a tyrannical force that affects five organs of the body. The five organs are:

Heart

Lungs

Kidney

Spleen

Liver

The yang organs are: six organs, which include:

Stomach

Large Intestine

Small Intestine

Gallbladder

Triple Burner

Bladder

The two essential elements of our bodies-blood and qi- could be represented in yin-yang. The body's life force is Yang in its nature, as it is vital, strong as well as continuous. Blood, on the contrary the other hand, is of a yin nature. It's a liquid that's rich in moisture, and nutritious.

It is further divided into five distinct phases of earth. They are:

Wood

Fire

Earth

Metal

Water

These five components are the human stages, that comprise:

Birth

Growth

Maturation

Death

Rebirth

In relation to these relationships In relation to these relationships, each of the organs known as yin-yang is connected to the fifth phase that make up the Earth.

The wood element is linked to the gallbladder, as well as the liver. The triple burner, the small intestine, as well as the heart are all related to fire. The stomach and the spleen are underneath Earth. The Metal component is responsible for the large intestinal tract and lung. Finally, Water relates to the kidneys and bladder.

Based on these relationships it is believed that when there is an imbalance of force in the body, and yin and Yang do not match Knowing which organ it is linked to will aid in diagnosing and treatment. The herbal medicine to treat this may be recommended for the appropriate patient.

The basis of TCM relies in the direction of being able to heal oneself. Man can harness his own power through the use of home remedies for self-healing. You are the only one who can manage your own health. Your choices affect only you and you are the only one accountable. Self-healing is the ideal type of treatment. Through the use of TCM it is possible to use additional techniques that allow the body to repair it self.

One of the biggest tasks for practitioners of Traditional Chinese Medicine is to recognize and appreciate the benefits of self-therapy. It is easy to become accustomed to Western medical practices that all else is not natural. It is logical. TCM is a treatment that employs distinct techniques and strategies. It might require time to get used to it, but the possibility that Traditional Medicine becoming a Universal Medicine is to be able to endure.

TCM employs five of the sensory parts of the human body (including the pulse) in order to pinpoint the root of an illness. In this instance, are considered to be related to imbalances in the qi and yin-yang force.

Chinese psychology is an additional component of TCM which helps to explain medical problems through instabilities of emotional health. If you're more depressed and the depressed you will be; this can affect your energy and Qi also negative. It could also have negative consequences. A different theory in Traditional Chinese Medicine is that the type of treatment that a patient receives depends on the beliefs they hold. The belief of a patient in the effectiveness of healthcare is vital for the treatment to function.

It is essential to have some form that trust exists between the patient and physician for treatment to be effective. The physician must make sure that they are aware of all aspects regarding the patient's health. There is no room for error in the event that they need to know the exact reason and a solution. There are times when patients might be cautious about the treatment employed for treating their ailments. If this is the case it is suggested to not have a doctor prescribe the remedy in question since it isn't useful.

Traditional Chinese Medicine is a therapy that is high-quality as well as, at time, at the same time affordable. The principles that are followed by TCM are a holistic treatment for ailments.

The Evolution of Chinese Medicine

The roots of Chinese treatment are thought to be a bit hazy. We believe that four distinct stages influenced the development of TCM. Four of these periods witnessed certain famous medical experts in the development of Chinese medical practice. Beginning with the time in the 29th Century BCE.

Phase One

The early period of the three, 4 Chinese rulers were deeply with medicine and had significantly contributed in the medical field.

Fu Xi, Shennong, and Huangdi were three of the most powerful ruling class.

Fu Xi introduced the world of medical science to Bagua The concept of which established the base for the concept of yin-yang. Organs in different bodies were judged as either yin or Yang and used to make more precise analysis.

Then followed Shennong who was infamously referred to as the father of Chinese Medicine and The Divine Husbandman. According to his name as the Red Emperor was believed to have developed the plow and played using plant medicines, classifying them into superior, medium as well as inferior.

Huangdi is the 3rd emperor and was also known as The Yellow Emperor. The legend says that he was been the most sophisticated of the three Emperors. He is the person who invented the acupuncture needles, which are nine in number. The medical techniques he developed were focused in the prevention of diseases and not their treatments.

The elements of the five earths were also influential in Chinese Traditional Medicine. It was believed that holistic relationships were linked to various organs in the human body. It was believed that Yin-yang is unevenly distributed throughout different organs.

Phase Two

Following the initial phase, there was an eminent doctor Bian Qiao whose contribution to Chinese medical practice are considered to be remarkable to date. Bian Qiao's history was documented about 2000 years following Huangdi. There appear to be a variety of legends regarding the existence of Bian Qiao in itself. There is a belief that Qiao's encounter using Chinese herbs helped him discover the mysteries of the human anatomy.

Numerous credits have been given to Bian Qiao, the magician who has been credited with his amazing healing abilities. The belief is that he can bring people back to their former lives applying Acupuncture. Bian Qiao was a remarkable doctor who believed in treating any disease as fast as it was possible prior to turning to be fatal. Bian Qiao was a doctor of science and strongly opposed the practice of superstition.

Phase Three

In the wake of Bian Qiao was the group of expertswho were Zhang Zhongjing, Hua Tuo, and Wang Shuhe. Zhang Zhongjing was a savant that was very attentive to physical signs and specifics. He was a keen observer and a lot of people were influenced by his virtue-based teachings throughout the 16th century. Zhongjing was honored by his incredible cure for Typhoid.

Hua Tuo was an obstetrician who had the ability for his use of anesthetics. It was uncommon at the time. He was a believer in simple yet effective treatment. His work with Chinese medicine has earned him the status of the most skilled Chinese surgeon in the world.

Another renowned figure in Chinese time included Wang Shuhe. Shuhe was a medical doctor recognized for his expertise in diagnosing. The accuracy of his diagnoses and treatment of any disease, relied on the pulse rate of patients. It was used by him to identify imbalances within the body. According to him, the pulse was a measure of all the energy that is present in the body.

Phase Four

China was hit by an outbreak of smallpox in this time. Unknown figures introduced populace to the technique of immunizing, and it resulted in reducing the death rate. The realm of Chinese medical practice has evolved significantly since the time.

Following the time of the emperors and doctors were over, the people started collecting the lessons of these men of great stature and wrote these down in various textbooks and the encyclopedias. Thus, the the traditional Chinese medical practices have come quite a ways with leaders, practitioners and physicians. While initially used only in China, TCM is now utilized as a healing tool by all across all over the world.

Each dynasty, and every rule, the medical world of China expanded and changed. Each of the rulers mentioned in the preceding paragraphs (and others) have been involved in the making of Traditional Chinese Medicine what it now. We've learned about the historical roots of Chinese medicine as well as the key people who played a significant role in its development. We now need to discover the therapies that comprise Traditional Chinese Medicine.

Types of TCM

Traditional Chinese Medicine has a deeply philosophical method of the healing process. It is a broad range of methods for treatment. The following are the various methods below:

Acupuncture

The treatment can be used to treat various conditions. It involves using needles placed through the body to pressure points to alleviate pain and resolve any other ailments. There are 2 000 pressure points within the body of a human. Acupuncture can be used to relieve neck pain, back tension, headaches or even respiratory ailments. It is a complex procedure, but it may as well provide very positive outcomes.

Acupressure

The treatment works similarly as acupuncture. However, it makes use of fingers and hands to push on your body's pressure points instead of needles. Meridians in the body are utilized to create a framework on where the therapy is executed.

Cupping

The method of cupping is unique which uses specific cups that can consist of any number of different materials. The cups are utilized to produce suction, and alleviate any pain in the body. They are usually warmed up in order to create suction across the surface of your skin. It is utilized as an approach to increase the flow of Qi throughout the body.

Cupping may also be utilized in cooperation to treat acupuncture in certain situations. It works by placing the needles over the points that are pressured and using the cup on top of the needles, completely covering them.

Moxibustion

This procedure is based on the combustion of leaves of mugwort near the site affected. The leaves are placed upon fire in close proximity to the skin in order to keep the heat. The smoke releases a strong smell that is almost unpleasant as well as smoke. Moxibustion, a remedy is believed to replenish Qi and improve the equilibrium of the yin and Yang throughout the body.

Meditation

It is a method of meditation that which you are likely to have heard of. It is a method of relaxing yourself and allowing yourself to be content with things around you is the primary objective of meditation. It is a process that has different significance for each person, however it's a highly beneficial method to protect yourself from illnesses. The key is tapping the positive energy that is stored within your. The breathing and meditation exercises are part in a broader category of therapies known as Qi Gong. The method of healing falls under TCM too.

Massage

Massage, also known as Tui Na can also be utilized to treat a Chinese Traditional treatment. The meridians in the body are utilized to locate the pressure points, and massaging them with great care. Ointments and oils are also commonplace in this type of therapy. This helps to relax body muscles, and eases physical as well as mental stress.

Herbal Therapy

Chinese herbal therapy is using Chinese herbal remedies to treat ailments. This is a complicated method of treatment that uses herbs in order to provide an effective treatment for various diseases. Chinese Herbal Medicine is the part in Traditional Chinese Medicine that we will explore in greater detail in this guide.

Medication and Non-Medication Therapies

Traditional Chinese Medicine separates the treatment options above into two categories. There are both medication and non-medical treatments. While both focus on self-healing, there are some distinctions that distinguish them. Acupuncture and similar therapies, where healing takes place as an actual physical process. It's a direct therapy which focuses on fixing the problem. The non-medical treatment is believed to be more simple and straightforward to apply.

However medications are comparable with herbal treatments. They're regarded to be more indirect in their way. It's a long and complex process to implement this type of treatment.

Chinese Herbal Medicine

The traditional Chinese Herbal Medicine uses the power of Chinese herbs to heal and regeneration. The herbal treatments aren't meant to heal illnesses generally. They are based upon the person who is taking them. Chinese herb therapy can be described as a method of treatment where the medication is developed by the body of the patient. An herbal remedy that is unique could be developed to suit a person's needs based on heartbeat, physical symptoms along with the other factors previously mentioned.

Chinese Herbal Medicine is based on the same foundations like Traditional Chinese Medicine. Qi is the principle of the yin-yang principle, and the harmony of forces all have roots deep within this therapy. Herbs are said to be equally efficient as traditional medicines. They're widely believed for having the same power as the pharmaceutical ingredients. It is for this reason that the treatment is now gaining popularity across the globe.

Chinese plants are believed to be beneficial and organic remedies to treat a variety of ailments. CHM is a sub-discipline of TCM however it's an extensive and complex universe in its own too. The world is now realizing the effectiveness and reliability of Chinese Herbal Medicine is. There's a lot of potential for many studies in TCM as well as CHM. If sufficient time and cash is devoted for research, the benefits for these treatments can be investigated in greater detail.

In CHM practitioners diagnose people with the help of pulse, symptoms and various other gauges. Another approach is to look at the color of the tongue as well as texture as well as dryness. This can help determine the strength and force of qi throughout the body. It is believed that in Chinese Herbal Medicine, the balance between yin and Yang is vital significance. If external and internal influences affect this state and cause instability which can cause the development of inflammation and diseases. CHM seeks to bring this equilibrium back to its initial condition, which is the same.

The medicine believes in the equilibrium of these two forces. It also believes in the balance of the qi. Health and mental well-being are associated through this harmony.

The History of Chinese Herbal Medicine

Chinese herbal remedies have been utilized to treat ailments since the beginning of time. The most well-known herbalist was Shennong which was an integral component of the growth of Chinese Herbal Medicine. He developed almost 365 remedies which helped people who worked employed in agriculture. The work of his is considered as the underlying morals behind the knowledge we have concerning Chinese Herbal Medicine today.

After we've gained a fundamental knowledge of the essence of Traditional Chinese Medicine is and what it does, we can look at what the benefits from Chinese Herbal Medicine are. The importance of making use of Chinese remedies.

Chapter 13: Why Use Chinese Medicine?

We've established a basic understanding of the nature of Chinese Traditional Medicine is, and now we'll look at what you can do with this method. TCM is utilized to treat various conditions or diseases such as asthma, allergies and even infertility. Through treatments such as Acupuncture and herbal therapy to restore balance, the body can be brought back.

When we are learning more about Chinese Herbal Medicine, it's crucial to be aware of the types of diseases it's able to with:

Cold and cough

Diabetes

Dementia

Liver issues

Insomnia

Menopausal symptoms

Stroke

Weight loss

Stress

and there are many more.

Herbal therapy is a straightforward treatment that addresses issues using energy. It's a means to reenergize your body.

How Does It Work?

Chinese Herbal Treatment works in 3 phases. It's a complete process that works on the basis of the natural laws. Each step is designed to fully heal the body and the mind.

Symptomatic Care

It is the initial stage of CHM. This program aims to discover and treat the symptoms of the patient. This initiative makes use of herbs to treat any abnormalities that patients suffer from. What is important to keep in mind is distinguishing between various symptoms, and classifying the condition of the patient. This is a crucial process because, depending on the patient's condition it will determine the best treatment to be prescribed.

Another aspect that is in consideration is that the state of mind and their thoughts must be taken into consideration. Prior to deciding on a method of treatment it is essential that the patient be informed about the previous.

Corrective Care

The third step of Chinese Herbal Medicine is to determine the exact cause(s) of manifestations in your body. Once the root cause is identified the procedure aims to eliminate the underlying cause at the root. Patients must be provided with treatment within a space in which they can feel safe and secure.

Prophylactic Care

It is the final phase of treatment. The goal is to improve the body's immune system after the illness is controlled. Strengthening the body and maintaining fitness is the prophylactic health's main goal.

Why Should You Use It?

One of the questions that comes up is the reason to use Chinese Herbal Medicine. The current state of society moment, we're eating artificially manufactured goods greater than we think is appropriate.

Pharmacological treatments may be the traditional method to treat the symptoms of an illness, however, it's the most unnatural method of fixing your body's health in the middle of your day. In addition, using pharmaceuticals for every single issue that you face can reduce its effectiveness to the body. It will lead to an increase in the dosage of these drugs and can cause further damage to the body.

Herbs are natural cures for all kinds of issues within the body. They are able to be utilized in various methods and provide favorable results that don't diminish your immune system or affecting your health in any manner. Herbal remedies have been proven to provide real-life results that improve your body's resistance. Improved performance, greater immune system, and improved levels of energy are only a few beneficial negative effects Chinese herbs are known to have.

Chinese Herbal Medicine is not only a method. It may be utilized in conjunction with various other treatments too. Acupuncture, meditation or Western medical are just a few ways of treatment CHM could be combined with. Combining several treatments in a combination can yield amazing outcomes.

Herbal therapies, or Traditional Chinese medicine in general provides a customized treatment plan for you. Contrary to western practices of healing which suggest that a specific condition can be dealt with by a particular method Chinese medical practices pay attention to the flow of energy within an individual, and recommends treatments based on that flow.

Instead of merely hiding or removing some symptoms Chinese Herbal Medicine focuses on giving complete healing to the body as well as the area affected by illness. The effectiveness of the herbal treatments is dependent on the individual, their condition and the body's immune system. A similar treatment can result in different results for various patients. Chinese Herbal Medicine is said to be individualized for every patient due to this.

Instead of prescribing generic medicines to treat every symptom, Chinese Medicine gives you an individual diagnosis that is tailored to the needs of your body just. Qi's presence and the balance of force, which is yin and Yang, are the primary tenets in

Traditional Chinese Medicine, and they give your body an opportunity to reenergize. Consuming only natural ingredients cause little or no harm to your body, and simultaneously, at the time, at the time helps restore the equilibrium of energy within one's body.

Herbal medicine will bring about positive change within one's daily life. In addition to helping help with ailments, but also treating yourself with natural remedies can help you feel more energetic, and also help to eliminate any minor problems that may be present in the body. The primary focus on Chinese Herbal Medicine is not only on the condition or the side effects. The goal is to treat the whole body. In the event of any energy issues or deficiencies, the herbs can help fix these.

Herbal remedies treat people with signs throughout the body. From the pulse to breathing patterns taking all factors into the mind of the doctor, an assessment can be made, and then the remedies are prescription-based. Sometimes, there's no treatment for a specific problem. When this happens, Traditional Medicine encourages the significance of quality of living. Instead of dwelling on the impossibilities or not being concerned about the longevity of a person, living quality is viewed as a valuable asset.

The way you live is a factor in determining your medical diagnosis. The way you eat, sleep cycle, activities such as movement and sleep are considered in the use of herbs for treatment. Certain herbal remedies may need to alter their diets or sleeping times. Every action you take has the ability to affect your qi. It is important to be positive and eat a healthy diet as well as exercise regularly for keeping your energy balance.

If you do not have any signs or symptoms, Chinese Herbal Therapy can aid in preventing these. If there is even the tiniest of irregularities such as the pulse of your body, a qualified practitioner will be able to alert you when something is amiss in the body. Chinese Herbal Medicine can further assist in relieving anxiety and help put your body at ease. It increases the circulation of positive energy throughout your body. This can allow you to feel calmer using herbal therapies.

Because Chinese Herbal Medicine works to stop diseases and infections It is a great opportunity to invest in. The prevention of disease from the start will, at any time far superior to treatment. Prior to the issue arising it is imperative to stop it off in its early stages. Thus, CHM can be useful in the future and contribute to the improvement of the global health system.

CHM concentrates on the prevention of or preventing illnesses. It promotes healing the mind, as physical treatments will only be effective when you are in a healthy and healthy body. Mind and body are in direct proportion to each other. Every one of them affects the health of the other. The primary energy source in the body is called qi and the energy working deep within you is known as vital qi. According to TCM's perspective Vital qi represents the very essence of you.

The concept behind CHM is to safeguard your qi in the core of your body that's the energy power of your entire body. The risk of a compromising circumstance wouldn't be a possibility if your Qi were safe and free from harm by external sources.

Cautionary Measures

Prior to beginning any type of herb-based medicine, you'll require the permission from your physician or doctor. It is not possible to mix the use of prescription drugs and herbs. Also, you must provide specific details about any prior or genetic diseases. The doctor will determine a suitable dosage of herbal medicine on your behalf based on the various factors. In the world, Traditional

Chinese Medicine is utilized in a variety of methods. But, in general TCM is employed for one of these motives:

Cultural and historical influences significantly influence the usage of herbs of a country. The country's history and growth within these regions can affect the herbology as well as other techniques influenced by culture.

A supplementation of herbal treatment is common in several nations. In addition to conventional treatments herbal therapy is also a element of therapy.

Every country can follow or implement Chinese Herbal Medicine in their individual way, according to their particular way of life.

The benefits from Chinese Herbal Medicine Another advantage that comes with making use of Traditional Chinese Medicine is the cost-effectiveness. It is possible to have a specialized procedure specifically tailored to your needs for a minimal cost. Even though TCM is considered as being on the same level with traditional medical practices and, most of the time it is only available when you're willing to shell out a large sum. That's why countries that are less developed could have greater use of traditional remedies compared to fully developed countries.

There are a number of benefits from Chinese Herbal Medicine, which will help us understand why it is worthy of being given the respect it deserves.

Personalized

Like we said earlier, CHM is a treatment that is unique to each patient. The symptoms and internal differences can affect the body's balance and lead to a distinct treatment for every patient. Every person has the body and qi forms, and also their own suitability. Each patient (even who share similar symptoms) might have their own diagnoses and prescribed.

Skin Healer

Chinese Herbal Medicine is extensively employed for the treatment of skin issues. For the cause of irritation, discoloration or other problems, CHM effectively treats numerous skin issues.

Energizer

Once you have started using Chinese Herbal Medicine in your life, you'll observe that you are driven to be more productive and that the energy levels of your are rising. It is because certain herbs provide an energy boost. The regular consumption of Chinese herbs will boost the mood of your body, lower stress levels and help you feel relaxed.

Eliminates Insomnia

The effects of insomnia can result in a major energy imbalance within the body. The problem isn't even addressed in a rapid manner. Chinese herbalism can be employed to treat insomnia and achieve an immediate 7-9 hours of sleep and not for lengthy therapy durations.

Rest and Digest

Herbs place the body into the parasympathetic state, which allows the body to ease into digestion and relax more effectively.

Fertility and Menstrual Problems

Infertility and menstrual disorders are treatable with Chinese Herbal Medicine. Issues like bleeding excessively throughout menstrual cycles could be effectively treated by CHM. Sexual problems in males as well as females can be treated.

www.ingramcontent.com/pod-product-compliance
Lightning Source LLC
Chambersburg PA
CBHW062139020426
42335CB00013B/1264